The Episode

The Episode

A True Story of Loss, Madness and Healing

Mary Ann Kenny

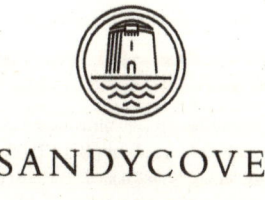

SANDYCOVE

an imprint of
PENGUIN BOOKS

SANDYCOVE

UK | USA | Canada | Ireland | Australia
India | New Zealand | South Africa

Sandycove is part of the Penguin Random House group of companies
whose addresses can be found at global.penguinrandomhouse.com

Penguin Random House UK,
One Embassy Gardens, 8 Viaduct Gardens, London SW11 7BW

penguin.co.uk

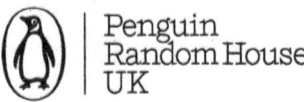

First published 2025

001

Copyright © Mary Ann Kenny, 2025

The moral right of the author has been asserted

Penguin Random House values and supports copyright. Copyright
fuels creativity, encourages diverse voices, promotes freedom
of expression and supports a vibrant culture. Thank you for purchasing
an authorized edition of this book and for respecting intellectual property
laws by not reproducing, scanning or distributing any part of it by any
means without permission. You are supporting authors and enabling
Penguin Random House to continue to publish books for everyone.
No part of this book may be used or reproduced in any manner for the
purpose of training artificial intelligence technologies or systems. In accordance
with Article 4(3) of the DSM Directive 2019/790, Penguin Random House
expressly reserves this work from the text and data mining exception

Set in 13.5/17.75pt Perpetua Std
Typeset by Jouve (UK), Milton Keynes
Printed and bound in Great Britain by Clays Ltd, Elcograf S.p.A.

The authorized representative in the EEA is Penguin Random House Ireland,
Morrison Chambers, 32 Nassau Street, Dublin D02 YH68

A CIP catalogue record for this book is available from the British Library

HARDBACK ISBN: 978–1–844–88686–9
TRADE PAPERBACK ISBN: 978–1–844–88687–6

Penguin Random House is committed to a sustainable future
for our business, our readers and our planet. This book is made from
Forest Stewardship Council® certified paper

This book is dedicated to the memory of my husband, John, and my mother, Bernadette (Bernie)

Contents

Author's Note ... ix

PART ONE: APRIL–DECEMBER 2015

1 Where's Dad? ... 3
2 May You Never ... 10
3 Is It Grief, or is It Depression? ... 21
4 On Fire ... 28
5 Crisis Assessment ... 41
6 Medication Madness ... 48
7 Asylum ... 65
8 Into the Abyss ... 76
9 Whether You Want It or Not ... 92
10 The Matter of My (Non-)compliance ... 106
11 Do They Like Colouring or Do They Like Lego? ... 110
12 Quarry ... 119
13 False Confession ... 129
14 Specialled ... 143
15 Metamorphosis ... 153
16 This Hospital Does Not Dispense Sweets ... 167
17 Supervised Visits ... 183

Contents

18 Safety Planning	192
19 Pink Armchair	203
20 Feedback	211
21 Basket Case	218

PART TWO: AFTERMATH

22 Minecraft Cake!	227
23 Is There Anything Else?	239
24 Summer Dress	249
25 I Know I Have Myself	258
Works Cited	271
Acknowledgements	273

Author's Note

There are two main sources for this book: my own memory, and records that I requested under the Freedom of Information Act from psychiatric services and from Tusla (the Child and Family Agency). These records provide a comprehensive and detailed account of what happened to me from the perspective of the two institutions. My electronic patient record alone runs to eight volumes and 875 pages, covering the entire three-year period of my involvement with the mental health service from my GP's referral in August 2015 to my last out-patient appointment in September 2018, while my Tusla file comprises 491 pages relating to the six-month period between October 2015 and March 2016.

Both sets of records provide an extremely rich source of information, right down to the detail of exactly what was said by me and others while I was being treated by psychiatric services and being assessed by Tusla. When quoting directly from written records, I employ the convention of using italics in combination with single inverted commas. When I narrate conversations with medical staff and social workers, I draw on the written records and on my personal memories of what was said. The written records of

Author's Note

conversations, though often extremely detailed, are not comprehensive transcripts, and in a small number of cases I draw on my memory alone to reconstruct something that was said as part of an exchange that is otherwise captured in my records; in such instances, I make it clear for the reader that this is what I am doing. Passing comments, small jokes and the odd personal detail shared with me by the professionals may be assumed by the reader to be based on my memory alone.

I have used pseudonyms throughout, employing inverted commas the first time each name occurs to signal that it is not the person's real name. The only names left unchanged are those of my husband, John, and my mother, Bernadette (Bernie).

PART ONE

April–December 2015

I

Where's Dad?

If my husband John had planned his death, he couldn't have scripted a more perfect scene. Bright spring sunshine. Out for a run in the crisp air on the granite hills of Killiney, the blue sweep of the bay stretching out in front of him, the coconut scent of flowering gorse. Fresh green shades of trees coming into leaf. The busy chatter of birds nesting. His favourite jogging playlist of fast tracks coming through his headphones. A few hours to himself to get his stay-at-home-dad life back on track, with the children at school and me at my lecturing job. Time to start a new fitness regime after a weekend socializing and the lingering chest cold of a long winter. As he left the house, stretching out his long, stiff limbs after squeezing past the red foliage of the overgrown forest flame in our front garden, John waved goodbye to a neighbour. She was the last known person to see him alive.

The first indication I had that something was wrong was when I glanced at my phone at around 1.45 p.m. and noticed six missed calls. I had just come out of a three-hour work meeting into the dazzling spring sunshine. It

The Episode

was a five-yearly programmatic review with an external panel of academics and representatives from industry, and it was of sufficient importance for me to have turned my phone off fully for the duration. As I strolled back towards my office building, chatting with colleagues, nodding a smiling 'hello' to students, and enjoying the feeling of warmth spreading through my body, I switched on my phone. In those days, my attitude to mobile phones bordered on dislike, and I had an old-fashioned button Nokia that I used mainly for text messaging. Receiving even one call on it was a rare occurrence, never mind six missed calls, and a small sense of alarm stirred deep inside as I squinted at the display. I hurried back to my office desk and Googled the two numbers that were visible, something I'd seen John do whenever he wanted to check the identity of a caller before ringing back. The first number was a local landline which threw up no results at all in Google; the second turned out to be St Michael's Hospital in Dun Laoghaire.

I had no idea why St Michael's would want to contact me, and I didn't have a name to call back, so I dialled the other number from which I had missed a call, the local landline. The secretary from my younger son's school answered and said that he hadn't been collected at pick-up time.

Next, I called the home phone, which rang out.

Then I called John's mobile. A man – not John – answered. He introduced himself as a garda.

Where's Dad?

'Something has happened to John,' he said. He told me to come to St Michael's and to bring somebody with me.

'What's happened to John?' I whispered.

Instead of answering my question, the policeman repeated his instructions.

Turning slowly to the colleague sitting at the desk next to mine, I gasped: 'Something has happened to John. I think he's dead.'

My colleague offered to drive me to the hospital. As we travelled around Dublin on the M50 towards Dun Laoghaire, I tried to figure out what might have befallen John. Initially I was thrown by the fact that a policeman had answered his phone, and I wondered had there been an accident, or had John been assaulted. Then I remembered the jog he had been preparing for that morning when I had called him from work at around 10 a.m., and I thought of his father dropping dead at the age of fifty-five and John's own fear that he too might die prematurely despite his apparently good health. So, when we reached the hospital and the same garda who had answered his phone informed me in the car park that John had collapsed and died during his morning run, he was confirming what I already suspected.

I was met at the hospital entrance by an old friend – I'll refer to him as 'K' – who lived nearby and who had jumped on his bike as soon as he received my call from my colleague's car. He and I were taken to identify the body. The staff who accompanied us there were kind and solicitous and

The Episode

approached me with an air of hushed reverence. Before entering the morgue, I was warned that the corpse would still be intubated and that several people would be in the room with me. Having identified John's body, we were then accompanied to a small office at the front of the building where I calmly went through everything else that was required of me.

I asked to view the body for a second time, this time on my own. Back in the morgue, I stared at John's bloodless face, unable to connect it with the happy smile beaming back at me at my fiftieth birthday party three days previously, where I had given a short impromptu speech in which I thanked John for our gorgeous children and our beautiful home and our perfect life together, almost as if I'd had a premonition of what was to come.

As I walked back along the corridor to where K was waiting, the hospital worker who accompanied me shared two pieces of advice. 'Find a funeral director as soon as possible to take care of the arrangements,' he urged me. 'And make sure you get the funeral *you* want.'

I didn't expect family strife over the funeral arrangements – in fact, it was the prospect of *minimal* family involvement that chilled me. John was an only child, and both his parents were dead. I came from a family of six, but all my siblings lived abroad.

'Is there some family nearby you would like to call?' I was asked when I returned from the morgue. I explained that my mother was elderly and hard of hearing, and that, although she was in good health for her ninety years, I would prefer to tell her in person. Then I used the hospital phone to call my brother in the UK, and he promised to be with me by evening.

The first time I cried was when I asked the hospital staff how I was to break the news to my children. While I don't recall their exact response, I do know that it contained the word 'heaven', and I remember the absolute certainty I felt that if there was one word I would not be using when I talked to my sons it was 'heaven'.

In an effort to delay as long as possible the moment when I would shatter my children's happiness, I suggested to K when we emerged into the blinding sunshine that we walk the pier in Dun Laoghaire. Once there, I stopped to call my younger sister in the States, where she would now be awake. Then I talked to the neighbour who was minding my sons, and I found myself overwhelmed by an urge to hold them in my arms.

The most terrible moment of that terrible day was telling the boys. Before meeting them, I had briefly entered our empty house, where John had left breakfast crumbs on the countertop in the kitchen and the water heater running for his post-jog bath. Then K and I walked the five minutes to my neighbour's house. It had been my intention to bring the children home to talk to them there, but as we made our way back, my older son kept interrogating me about his

The Episode

father's whereabouts. 'Where's Dad?' he asked me over and over. 'I'll tell you when we get home,' I kept repeating. 'Is he dead?' he asked me finally, stopping me in my tracks. Aged only eight, he had always been wiser than his years. I have a memory of the three of us standing immobilized in the middle of the road. K was there too, but he doesn't feature in the scene where the sun is glaring down on us, the children are wailing in anguish, and I am repeating over and over, 'I'm sorry, I'm sorry,' an expression I used with other people that day too, as if I was blaming myself for the devastation they were feeling.

I don't remember much about the evening. I had asked K to contact my mother and to drive her to our house so I could tell her in person. 'Don't cry, boys,' she instructed as we all sat together in our sitting-room, and I snapped back at her that they could cry if they wanted to. She was just as bewildered as everyone else, but she angered me at that moment with her old-fashioned, schoolteacher-ish directives, so familiar to me from my childhood, when our needs had always seemed less important than those of the adults in our lives. 'And don't speak to me in Irish in front of them,' I added, furious that she was attempting to give me coded messages about my children while they looked on helplessly, struggling to make sense of the tragedy that had befallen them.

Years later I would read that what we call madness often begins with 'normal' cognitions and 'normal' emotions. I believe that the roots of the pathological guilt I suffered in the second half of 2015 can be found in the events of 21 April, when I assumed full and sole responsibility for shattering my children's lives because I was the one to disclose to them that their father was dead. But the details of the day John died would not appear anywhere in the voluminous files that were created about me and my family later that year by psychiatric services and by Tusla, the national Child and Family Agency. Of all the mental health and child-protection professionals to interact with me in the months following John's death, only one would ever ask me to talk about the events of 21 April 2015, and that was the therapist I visited directly afterwards, long before I ever broke down.

2

May You Never

I got the funeral I wanted – and that John would have wanted. The mood was celebratory and defiant, and more than half of the Humanist service in the packed Victorian Chapel at Mount Jerome Crematorium in central Dublin was given over to music. I got the idea of making song a central part of the service from the way John had organized his own mother's funeral five years earlier, when a favourite track of his had been played as part of a Protestant service that was much more personalized than the Catholic funeral masses I was used to. I recalled the intensity of listening to music in the company of other mourners, in silent contemplation of my mother-in-law's life and death, and of being moved to tears by the lyrics of 'After Summer Rain' by the folk singer Steve Tilston, who was a personal friend of John's and had played at our wedding. 'There is much to treasure in what this moment brings,' Tilston sings, 'for there are always winds of change waiting in the wings.'

So I had 'After Summer Rain' played for John in the Victorian Chapel, along with another of Steve Tilston's songs,

'Sometimes in This Life'. Music wasn't just one of John's many interests, as a friend from his teenage years in Chester would tell the mourners when he addressed us in his eulogy; it was part of his character and part of his outlook on life. Several old friends of John's had told me unprompted and independently of one another in the days leading up to the funeral that when they thought of him, what came to mind was UK singer John Martyn's ode to friendship, 'May You Never'. So we listened to 'May You Never' and reflected on the centrality of friendship in John's life, especially as he'd had no siblings of his own. John Martyn was one of John's musical heroes and, by a strange coincidence that only struck me later, he was also sixty when he died in Ireland in 2009 and his body was also cremated in Mount Jerome. The last piece we listened to was Martyn's 'Bless the Weather', a haunting song about love and loss with a long instrumental piece in the middle that rang out into the high vaulted wooden ceilings of the chapel and gave us pause to feel deeply the acute pain of John's absence.

  I wanted the funeral service to be a celebration of John's life and to embody the theme of survival, not least because my children needed a message of hope. The eulogies were delivered by my middle brother on behalf of my family, and by a lifelong friend of John's from Chester who asked me in advance if it was OK to use humour, because John always made him laugh. I readily agreed, and as well as song, laughter was the other distinctive quality of the service that people

The Episode

would remember later. We heard many examples of John's ability to see the absurd humour in every situation, and my brother talked warmly about how John had enlivened the otherwise somewhat silent gatherings of our family. I sat back and allowed myself to be entertained by stories of the funny and rebellious man who had shared my life for fifteen years, watching my children's faces closely for their reactions as tributes were paid to John as an inspiring French teacher, a much-loved friend and a devoted father who had introduced them to the music of 'Uncle Frank Zappa' and 'Uncle Warren Zevon'. I chose not to speak publicly myself, and I asked the celebrant to read out the words of Bob Dylan's 'Death is Not the End' on my behalf.

I had never really understood the function of a large Irish funeral until I and my children became chief mourners. I was overwhelmed by the huge turnout of family, friends, neighbours, colleagues, children, their parents, school principals, teachers, and people I'd worked with twenty years previously and hadn't seen since. After the service, tears mixed with laughter as we took shelter from the sudden hail shower that seemed to have been waiting to assault us as we exited the chapel, and a large crowd adjourned to the warm, spacious tearooms at Mount Jerome, where the children mingled happily with their friends, and I felt surrounded by love and support. Later that evening, a smaller, more intimate group gathered in the bar of our local hotel and had a drink to John's memory.

Then the funeral was over, and everything stopped. My younger sister departed for her home in the States, having stayed in our house for ten days, and my brothers also dispersed to their lives abroad. The children returned to school. I had been advised to resume their regular routine as soon as possible, and while the older boy was reluctant to leave my side, the younger actually asked to go back to school and only ever missed one or two days during this period. I was lucky, at least initially, that my academic year was over, so there was no need for me to go to work, and the small amount of exam correcting I had to do could be completed from home. I achieved a lot in those early weeks – like changing my will to ensure it named guardians for my children in the event that something happened to me, and gathering up all the documentation needed for probate purposes by our family solicitor – and I also had lots of visitors. Yet my enduring memory of that time is one of inertia, of sitting immobilized in the sunroom at the back of a silent house filled with frozen dinners and fading white flowers, waiting for the children to come home from school while gazing out at the climbing clematis on the back wall of our garden as it came into pink flower and gradually withered away.

People always use metaphors to describe grief. For me it was like being knocked down by a speeding bus. It came out of nowhere and completely floored me. The most distinctive and least expected quality was physical. My hair didn't turn grey overnight as happens in novels (and sometimes in real

The Episode

life), but I lost my appetite and had difficulty sleeping, and my menstrual cycle, normally regular and predictable, went haywire. I spent most of the time bleeding and I remember three cycles within a short six-week timespan immediately following John's death. If ever proof were needed of the unity of body and mind, my reaction to the loss of John was it, and I was gripped by an excruciating pain that permeated my whole existence.

Almost as soon as he died, I stopped doing all the things that gave me pleasure: jogging, working, reading fiction, drinking alcohol, learning piano, listening to music, going out with friends, eating for pleasure, following chat shows on Irish radio. I avoided any place where we had been together. I hated crowds and I hid away from the ruthless glare of the spring sunshine. When I wasn't busy with paperwork or with the children, I sat in the armchair overlooking the back garden and reflected on the devastation of our lives. I thought about how my sons had lost so early one of the two people who loved them most in the world. They would have no male role model as they went through their teenage years unless someone – and I couldn't think who that might possibly be – stepped up to the mark. Nobody would ever tell them about the drama of attending their births or exactly how it was that John had ended up knocked out stone cold on the hospital floor while I was pushing our second baby out – just like his father at John's own birth. Nobody would be able to give the children an accurate account of John's family history, of the miners who had moved from Lancashire to work in North Wales, or exactly which relative was killed in the Battle of the Somme, or what the connection of John's grandma had been to the couple who witnessed the Phoenix Park murders in 1882. John had no family left, apart from a few distant cousins in the UK.

My own siblings had all moved abroad, most of them as long ago as the 1970s and 1980s. My mother lived nearby, and I was close to her, but she was extremely elderly and absorbed in the busyness of her own life, and wasn't, I felt, fully attuned to the emotional needs of my sons. I believed myself to be utterly alone and I felt crushed by the weight of responsibility for my children's very survival, as sole custodian of their physical, emotional, intellectual, social and mental well-being then and on the long road to adulthood.

While the boys were at school, I tried to help myself. I was desperate to find something to make me feel better, and I went for long walks in the neighbourhood, retracing John's final running route, past our neighbours' houses, under the cut-granite archway traversing Victoria Road, following the downhill curve of the road along the ivy-clad perimeter wall of Killiney Hill Park, and stopping at the gates of Ayesha Castle. In a secret, pain-filled ritual, I would place minuscule bunches of bluebells and sprigs of white, pink and red valerian picked at the roadside inside the narrow mock arrow slit above the spot where he had collapsed and died. When my mother was home, I would drop in to her house and crawl

The Episode

into bed, craving the oblivion of sleep in the room with the breathtaking sea views where I had spent time recovering from a miscarriage ten years previously. Sleep never came, and she would make tea for me like she had always done when I was ill. Then she would take my face in her hands, hold her eyes level with mine, and repeat to me over and over that I *would* eventually recover and that I *would* be happy again.

I read lots of books about bereavement and grieving. My shelves filled up with self-help books with titles like *Grieving Mindfully*; *Grieving: A Beginner's Guide*; and *Seven Choices: Finding Daylight after Loss Shatters Your World*. I didn't find much to identify with in those books, but reading them was a distraction, especially as I found it impossible to focus on any other subject. I looked for titles about widowhood, with or without young children, and found *Widow to Widow*, and *Death . . . And How to Survive It*. I was told about Sheryl Sandberg, who was chief operating officer at Facebook and the mother of two young children when, on 1 May 2015, just ten days after John's death, her husband died suddenly from heart-related causes during a gym workout. Thirty days later, Sandberg posted an essay on Facebook, and many people mentioned it to me, pointing out the similarities between her story and mine. I read the essay and wondered how anyone could claim to take stock of what they had learned through coping with loss a mere thirty days after the bereavement – even if, as Sandberg explains, this marks the end of intense mourning in the Jewish tradition. When tragedy strikes, Sandberg writes in her post, you have a choice: 'You can give in to the void. [. . .] Or you can try to find meaning.' I felt bad about giving in to the void and at the same time aggrieved at the suggestion that it was a *choice* I had made, or that meaning could possibly emerge so soon.

From mid-May, I visited a therapist once a week in his rooms nearby. 'Michael' was an elderly gentleman who came recommended by one of the parents in my younger son's school, and he would always prepare tea for us when I arrived. I'd never been for therapy before, so I wasn't sure what to expect. The best thing about those sessions was that he made me laugh and that, for a brief interlude, the agony would recede. Michael had an infectious laugh and a grandfatherly air about him, and I remember him laughing both with and about me.

To begin with he asked me to describe my birth family and my place within it, before suggesting I might like to talk about John and how he had died. Mostly we discussed my fears for the future. I told him I was afraid that something might happen to me and that my children would be left alone, and he asked me to reflect on the likelihood of that happening. I discussed my worries about their future happiness, questioning my ability to parent them successfully alone into adulthood. Michael urged me not to view parenthood as a pre-programmed, monolithic block with the ability to crush me. Most of what we do as parents is reactive, he explained. We react to opportunities that arise in our children's lives and in ours, as we navigate our way through the various challenges and obstacles as best we can. He urged me to read *The Optimistic Child* by Martin Seligman, an American psychologist and founder of the positive psychology movement, so I ordered the book on Amazon, and we discussed Seligman's techniques for raising children to mastery and optimism.

I always left Michael's therapy rooms feeling a little better, but the weak spark of hopefulness invariably burned itself out within an hour or two. Apart from visiting my mother and being with the children, the only other source of comfort in that early period was spending time with friends. They would arrive after work with food to cook and small gifts for my sons and a DVD for later on, and they often stayed in the guest room overnight. There were three friends in particular who lived and worked locally and kept showing up with offers of support – K, his wife 'D', and another mutual friend, 'R', whom we had known since we had all lived in Germany together twenty-five years previously. I also had visits from abroad: a close friend in Berlin travelled to Dublin three times during that period, as did my UK-based brother. Lots of children came to the house, too. When parents from the schools my children were attending would ask how they could help, I told them to drop their kids over, so my sons would have the distraction of play, and I could watch wistfully from the kitchen window as they bounced happily on the trampoline or jostled each other on the slide and climbing frame crammed into the small garden at the rear of our house.

The parents at my older son's school helped in other ways too. In an inspired act of kindness, they organized a dinner roster to run until the end of the school term, and twice or three times a week until late June, my evening meal was delivered to me at home. They had offered to cook for the children too, but my older son especially would only eat food prepared by me. On days when a delivery was due, I would look forward to discovering what was on the menu; sometimes there'd be dessert and once even a bottle of chilled white wine. The only flaw in the arrangement was the loneliness of eating my dinner-for-one. So, when a mother announced one evening that instead of delivering a meal, she was inviting us to eat at hers, I gratefully surrendered all three of us to the warm, happy commotion of her kitchen and her family life. I needed more of other people's houses, and the best times of all were when we were invited once a week to stay over at the beautiful, welcoming home of my friend K, who had dropped everything to be with me the day John died, where we could briefly escape from the haunting memories and cold emptiness of our own house.

The children seemed OK most of the time, but my younger son adopted a high-pitched baby voice when interacting with adults – and with me in particular – while his older brother's nights were tormented. He howled for ten

The Episode

nights in a row immediately following John's death, and weeks later his sleep was still troubled. I lay beside him, thinking that his pain and my inability to soothe him at a time when I was barely able to function myself were the nearest thing to torture I was ever likely to experience. All I could do was hold him tight and echo my mother's words, telling him over and over that one day he would feel better and that we would all find happiness again. At times like that, I wished all four of us had died on 21 April. I wasn't suicidal, I just wished that we hadn't survived, and that my children especially had been spared the terrible suffering of grief.

3

Is It Grief, or is It Depression?

By late June, my siblings began to ask me over the phone if I thought I might be depressed and whether I believed that medication could help. My instinctive reaction to both questions was to say, 'No, I don't think so.' But I was frightened by the possibility of depression. Michael, my therapist, had urged me to be vigilant about diet and sleep, especially when I told him that I was losing weight and when I described the restless nights I spent wedged in between the sleeping forms of my two children. I relayed my siblings' concerns to him, and he was very firm that my presentation in our sessions together did not suggest depression to him.

'It's grief,' he told me. 'But, if you don't eat properly and make sure to get enough sleep, you'll end up depressed. And we need to avoid that.'

The question of whether I was clinically depressed two months after John's death, or whether what I was experiencing was 'normal' grief, goes to the heart of debates within and about psychiatry. There is little doubt that by early summer 2015, I was suffering from many of the symptoms

The Episode

commonly associated with depression: reduced appetite, weight loss, sleeplessness, fatigue, loss of pleasure, poor concentration, and low mood most of the day nearly every day. Small tasks seemed insurmountable and larger plans ended up being abandoned. I remember the enormous effort it took to get photos developed for my younger son's school project and to buy a bike for his older brother and transport it home in the back of my car. Meanwhile, the trip I had booked for early July to visit my brother in the US, along with the attic conversion planned for the summer months of 2015, proved too much for me to implement, especially when faced with my older son's staunch resistance to flying or travelling anywhere far from home or indeed to change of any kind. I also found myself unable to start making preparations for a return to work in early September, when the new academic year would start. The closer it came, the more I fended off my friends' offers of help with the important task of finding a childminder, not because I didn't want to, but because I wasn't able.

    I also struggled at this time to reflect on the past and on the substance of what I and the children had lost. When I tried to conjure up what John had looked like, I could remember back no further than the funeral parlour in the days following his death, when I had stared at his ashen face, trying to figure out what was different, until I realized that the three-day beard he had always worn had been shaved off and his mouth set in a pompous expression that was utterly

Is It Grief, or is It Depression?

out of character for the unpretentious, irreverent and affectionate man who had shared my life for fifteen years. Every afternoon, my younger sister would ring me from the States and I would cry down the phone, unable to summon up any memories of John when he was alive or of the happy years we had spent together. Even at the time, my inability to connect with life before his death struck me as odd. I was in the grip of an ice-cold, existential fear that centred around my responsibilities for my children. Worry and panic prevented me from confronting and integrating memories of the past or deriving any comfort from glimpsing the contours of 'Option B' – Sheryl Sandberg's term, in her book of the same name, for the alternative life we're forced to live when death has robbed us of our Option A.

But does any of this mean that I was suffering from a mental illness that required medication? Reactions to bereavement are occasionally pathological, necessitating medical intervention, but my therapist didn't think I was clinically depressed, and I wasn't experiencing the more severe symptoms of depression, like feelings of worthlessness and extreme guilt (these would come later). Furthermore, the little I knew about psychiatric drugs at that time made me doubt that they could be of benefit to me in my distress. I was aware that antidepressants are not just 'happy pills' and that they work by altering the chemistry of the brain in some way, and I was nervous of any substance that had the potential to change my mental state in ways I could not predict.

The Episode

'There's no shame in taking medication,' my siblings told me.

'Well, I'm not actually ashamed,' I said.

'If you're not keen on antidepressants,' they said, 'you could try a small amount of Xanax to take the edge off the pain.'

It wasn't *shame* that I felt when we had these conversations, but *fear* at the unknown effects of the pills. I discussed the matter with Michael, and he insisted that I did not need antidepressant medication, although he did suggest that a short course of sleeping tablets might help. My GP took the same position in early July as she wrote up a prescription for zopiclone, a sedative used for short-term treatment of insomnia. 'It's better, if you can, to get through grief without medication,' she advised when I cried to her about the unrelenting pain. 'And you won't thank me later if you become addicted to a drug like Xanax.' Not only did I not need a benzodiazepine or any other kind of psychiatric medication, she explained, but it could interfere with the grieving process by dulling the intensity of emotions that are important and necessary for the processing of loss.

I was content enough to accept the advice of the professionals, especially as my preference was to try to get by without medication. Even taking zopiclone for insomnia filled me with apprehension: I feared not waking in the night if a knock came to the front door or if the children needed me, and I worried that I might never be able to fall asleep naturally again if I developed a dependency on sleeping pills. In the end, I took them only a handful of times. The experience was fear-filled and resulted in only a marginal improvement in my sleep.

When I relayed Michael's comments about depression and medication back to my brother in the US, he urged me to find a CBT therapist. Cognitive behavioural therapy, or CBT, is a type of talking therapy based on the idea that at the root of depression are 'incorrect' judgements and 'distortions' of reality. I mentioned to Michael that we might need to look at CBT, and he laughed back at me, asking what it was I thought that we'd been doing in our sessions together.

Based on what I have since read and learned, I can now see the influence of CBT on the eclectic approach he took to the therapeutic situation with me. He challenged my negative thinking and encouraged me to write down my thoughts and feelings, especially when they were keeping me awake at night. He urged me to plan pleasurable activities, including the short trip to Galway we undertook as a family with his encouragement in early July. He asked me to describe the meals and menus I had previously enjoyed, and together we compiled a shopping list of the ingredients I would need to prepare some nice dishes for myself. He explained the 'Urgent–Important Matrix' to me, a simple tool to help prioritize a to-do list based on the urgency and importance of each task. And he encouraged me to use progressive muscle relaxation, deep breathing and other mindfulness techniques to distract myself from anxious thoughts.

The Episode

Michael had told me early on in our interactions that he would be taking a few weeks' holiday from the middle of July. This meant he would not be around during the family visit planned for later that month to celebrate my mother's ninetieth birthday. She had turned ninety in April, just eleven days before John died. The family party had always been scheduled for July and there had never been any question of cancelling, although I had wondered silently in the early days how it could possibly go ahead. As the time grew closer, Michael asked how I felt about his impending absence, and I assured him that I would have the support of my family while he was gone.

Much later, towards the end of 2015, I would often wish that I could turn the clock back to early July, to a time when I still had control over my mind and my body and when the worst problem I faced was the terrible agony of grief. To this day, I wish I could offer words of comfort and advice to my July 2015 self. I would urge myself not to fight or question the pain. I would tell myself that I *would* recover, but not to expect recovery too soon. I would share what I have since read about depression as a label for what is otherwise called 'sadness' or 'distress'. I would repeat to myself the words of English paediatrician and psychoanalyst Donald Winnicott, who described 'the capacity to become depressed, to have a reactive depression, to mourn loss' not as an illness, but as 'an achievement of healthy emotional growth'. I would

Is It Grief, or is It Depression?

encourage myself to find something that made me feel physically better, like a dance class or a ball sport involving other people, and to ditch the long, solitary, miserable walks that took me past the walls of Ayesha Castle where John had died.

I think I grieved 'too hard' in the months following John's death. Freud described the grieving process as 'Trauerarbeit', or 'grief work'. This is the notion that the bereaved must work through powerful feelings in order to break ties with the deceased, to adjust to new circumstances and to begin to build new relationships. Grief for me was like attempting to swim during a storm surge. I threw myself headfirst into it, without a life jacket or any other buoyancy aid. There were multiple reasons why things happened this way: the suddenness of John's death; the closeness of our relationship; the lack of immediate family support; the needs of the children and my strong identification with their suffering; and other aspects of my personality, like my impatience, my perfectionism, my realism and my lack of religious belief. Grieving this way took a heavy toll, but it may actually have been effective in the long run: I will never know whether it was the grief work I undertook in the early months or the shock at what happened later, but by the end of 2015 all the grief would be spent, and I would finally be ready to embrace my own 'Option B'.

4

On Fire

The party for my mother took place in Rosslare on 25 July 2015. It was the largest gathering of my immediate family since my father's death eleven years previously, with all six siblings assembled in one place for only the second time since the late 1980s. They arrived from abroad during the first half of July, accompanied by spouses and children; some stayed with my mother, some in rented accommodation nearby, and my older sister occupied the guest room in our house in the days leading up to the party weekend. She had been unable to travel from her home in New Zealand for the funeral in April, and when we met, she took me in her arms and I burst into tears. I reacted in a similar fashion on encountering my siblings' spouses and children, who were also meeting me and my sons for the first time since before John's death and funeral.

The celebratory dinner was a beautiful and fitting tribute to my mother, in a hotel chosen by her for the spectacular artwork on the walls, the beach a few short metres away, and the friendly staff who knew her from previous visits and were guaranteed to give us a warm welcome. I wore the same elegant black party dress with the pink floral print that I had treated myself to for the fiftieth birthday celebration in April and that I had worn for a second time just over a week later at John's funeral, almost as an act of defiance. Now the dress fitted me better because I was thinner. My sons sat at the grandchildren's table with their seven cousins, horse-playing their way through the meal, while I was quietly and cruelly aware of John's absence at what was otherwise a joyous occasion. When it came to speeches, we had decided collectively that each of my mother's six children would speak in turn. We took the floor in order of age. When it came to me, the second youngest, I thanked my mother with a shaking voice and my eyes brimming with tears for her loving support of me and the children since John's death three months earlier. 'You spoke very nicely,' my middle brother commented later that evening, 'and you're looking lovely.' I was touched by the rare words of tenderness in a family not versed in overt expressions of intimacy.

Over the party weekend, I took some Xanax for the first time. A few days beforehand, I had paid another visit to my local medical centre. Once again, I had asked tentatively about the advisability of antidepressants, and once again, my GP had recommended that we hold back on them, at least for the present. She was reluctant to agree to any medication, but I left her office with a prescription for Xanax. The drug came with a strong health warning: it was a highly

The Episode

addictive benzodiazepine, the doctor explained, and was to be used sparingly and only when I felt unable to cope otherwise. 'You can cut a pill in two if you don't want to take the full dose,' someone advised me in Rosslare. I hadn't known that you could do that with tablets, so I did as suggested and swallowed a minuscule amount of the drug for the first time. The experience was one of almost instant calming, tinged with fear that this was to be the first step towards dependency.

I also took my first sea swim of the year on Rosslare Strand that weekend, while my younger sister looked on. Afterwards I sat with her by the water's edge.

'That was fantastic!' I raved, as we gazed out together at the perfectly still light-blue expanse.

'You know, that's the first time I've heard you being enthusiastic about anything since I've come home,' she responded.

Sea-swimming has always been a passion of mine. I experience it as a form of natural therapy, and it was an enthusiasm that I shared with my mother, who continued to swim well into her eighties and whose smiling word 'afterglow' perfectly captured the lingering elation that always followed the dips we took together in the icy waters of the Irish Sea. If I could return to the months following John's death now, I would do lots of sea-swimming. I believe that the afterglow might have helped me to rediscover the joy of being alive.

*

On Fire

After the party weekend, when my siblings began to depart for their lives overseas, I experienced a rising sense of panic at the scale of what I needed to achieve before I could resume my job in early September. I had held a vague hope in the weeks leading up to the family visit that I would be offered practical help with the ever-lengthening to-do list on my fridge door. I had envisaged sitting down with one of my siblings and methodically working through the tasks, ticking them off one by one. But I had never voiced the expectation, and no one had proposed it in the busy schedule of family outings and social get-togethers. The most pressing issue was to find a childminder, and my younger sister had advised me to post a notice in the local shop. I hadn't acted on her suggestion, though, not because I didn't think it was a good idea, but because I felt unable to field the calls that would inevitably follow and to vet the candidates.

On 31 July, the day before my younger sister left for her home in the States, she suggested we visit my GP together. I no longer felt able to fend off the well-meaning suggestions of friends and family members that I try an antidepressant. We were met at the medical centre by a friendly young locum who responded that he could certainly write up a prescription if this was what I wanted, but that what I was experiencing was a bereavement reaction with understandable anxiety and depressive symptoms. I remember he took out a pen and wrote down the various factors that would contribute to my eventual recovery.

The Episode

'You *will* get better,' he assured me, 'with or without medication.'

He pointed at the list of words on his page. 'Social support will help. Plus exercise. Good diet. Plenty of sleep. And even the passage of time. There's certainly a place for medication too if that's what you'd like.'

'Yes, I might like to try that too,' I responded, and he wrote out a prescription for a daily dose of 50mg of sertraline.

'It's an SSRI,' the doctor explained. 'It increases serotonin levels in the brain and it works for depression. If you find it helpful, you could take it for a period of three to four months.'

'OK,' I said, hoping that I *would* find it helpful and that I wouldn't need to take it for any longer than that. *Maybe it will get me over the worst of the pain*, I thought, while also recalling my GP's advice that grief has to be worked through and that taking medication only postpones the inevitable agony.

'There may be side-effects,' the doctor cautioned, interrupting my thoughts. 'And you may feel worse before you start to feel better.' The pharmacist who filled the prescription later that afternoon said the same thing, and I was alarmed at the prospect of feeling worse than I already did. I also knew from everything else I had heard about antidepressants that they could take a number of weeks to take effect, and that even then, they might not work for me at all.

*

On Fire

I waited for more than twenty-four hours before starting the drug, agonizing over whether it was advisable at all, and fearing an adverse reaction while alone in the house with my children. Before going to bed on the evening of Sunday, 2 August, I took the prescribed dose for the first time. Some hours later, I awoke in a state of severe agitation. I was drenched in sweat, weak with nausea, and my legs and arms were prickling all over. I spent hours tossing in bed, gripped by terror. When morning came, I waited in anguish for my older sister to arrive. She was the only member of my family still in the country (my mother had left for a week-long poetry workshop in the UK), and she was due to depart for New Zealand later that week. In a foretaste of all the reactions I would experience from everyone I implored to help me over the following weeks, she stared back at me blankly as I attempted to communicate the agony of what I was experiencing.

It was a bank holiday Monday, and my local medical centre was closed, so I took the two doses of sertraline prescribed for the day, taking hope from the words I remembered from both doctor and pharmacist that I might feel worse before I started to feel better. The excruciating and persistent burning under my skin made it impossible for me to focus on the practical tasks that had to be tackled while my sister was out with the children. I recall needing to pay a motorway toll on her behalf, a task that took all my powers of concentration to achieve during the hours I spent alone in the house that afternoon.

The Episode

First thing Tuesday morning, I returned to the medical centre, where I met the same locum for a second time. '*In again*,' his notes from the appointment state, '*anxiety with sertraline* [. . .], *paraesthesia* [a painful tingling or prickling], *feels extremely anxious*'. He also noted that we had '*a long chat about controlled breathing and relaxation*'.

'I've decided to stop the medication,' I told the doctor.

'That's a wise choice,' he agreed. 'You'll feel better once the effects are out of your system.'

'We're due to fly to France in two days' time. I'm wondering whether the trip is a good idea at all.'

'You should go. And if necessary, we can revisit the antidepressants when you come back. Take the Xanax and the sleeping tablets with you and don't hesitate to use them if you feel the need while you're away.'

The children and I had received multiple invitations to spend time away during the summer months – from friends and family in Galway, the UK, Berlin and the US. When the French-Irish couple John and I had befriended through our children suggested that we spend a week with them in their second home in south-central France, I was attracted by the prospect of rest for me and companionship for the children. In the few remaining days until our departure on 6 August, I struggled to take care of the boys and prepare for our flight to Lyon while battling waves of perspiration and nausea and the persistent stinging sensations scorching my body. Even the simplest task, like packing bags or printing boarding cards or buying gifts for the French children, required extraordinary levels of effort. My three close friends arrived at the house again, asking how they could help, and R drove us to the airport. She would tell me later of her dismay at seeing the haunted look in my eyes and at realizing that I had made no progress at all during the weeks of the family visit.

Of the week I spent with my children in France in August 2015, my abiding memory is of lying on a bed in a darkened room, suffering from the oppressive heat, willing my body to recover. It was only with great difficulty that I was able to eat or sleep or focus on anything other than the stinging sensations. I swallowed the occasional half-tablet of Xanax or zopiclone, and when I did, I experienced a little relief and even managed to get some sleep. But the beneficial effects of the drugs only convinced me that I was developing an addiction, and I was gripped by a terrifying belief that soon I would not be able to function at all without medication. As I reclined in the dark, my limbs ablaze and my mind obsessing, I could hear my children playing outside with their friends, or occasionally squabbling over my iPad in the room next to mine. To this day, the frantic theme song of the Angry Birds game that seemed to be playing on a never-ending loop conjures up the intense heat and agitation of those hours.

As the week wore on, I made increasingly frantic calls to family and friends and to my local medical centre at home. I talked to my regular GP, who advised me to take the Xanax

The Episode

for anxiety and a sleeping tablet if it helped, and not to worry while I was away about the addictive potential of the drugs. I repeatedly phoned my friend R in Dublin, who encouraged me to try physical exercise and not to cut the holiday short. I also Skyped my brother in the US on a daily basis. He was insistent that what I was experiencing had nothing to do with the effects of the antidepressant, which in any case had now been expelled from my body.

'It's a stress reaction,' he explained, and he urged me to relax and to breathe deeply. 'You *will* get better,' he continued, 'but you need to *believe* that, not least for the children's sake.'

As I lay on my bed in the shaded room, I felt a crushing sense of failure at my inability to recover despite understanding that my children's happiness depended on it. I tried to focus on my breathing, to inhale deeply and to exhale slowly. But nothing could distract me from the excruciating prickling that engulfed my limbs and settled in a tight vice around my torso and my head. My brother had sent me web links explaining the physical effects of stress, and I read up on paraesthesia, learning that the painful tingling can also be caused by damage to peripheral nerves. The burning had persisted despite stopping the drug, so it seemed clear to me that the sertraline had caused permanent nerve damage, and I was convinced that I would never recover.

I was aware that the holiday was my one opportunity to find some respite from the trauma and exhaustion of the previous months, and I was desperate for rest. But I also felt guilty for being a bad house guest, and fearful of appearing lazy or ungracious or as wallowing in self-pity since John's no-longer-so-recent death. I reproached myself for taking a back seat with food preparation and with organizing the children's activities, and I tried hard to present a 'normal' front when we went on excursions or gathered around the huge outdoor dining table for yet another extended meal, with fresh rounds of the large French family arriving every day. I felt sharp pangs of envy, on both my own and my children's behalf, at the noisy gatherings of grandparents, aunts, cousins and in-laws who would embrace each other warmly and sit together chatting long after the children had gone to bed. My French friend had told me that if anything were to happen to her Irish husband, she would move back to her parents' home with her four children, and I secretly coveted the security and comfort of the safety net laid out on display in front of us.

Eventually the week in France came to an end. As we made our way through the airport in Lyon, I struggled to keep track of gate numbers, boarding cards and departure times. On the plane, the children bumped against me in the normal rough-and-tumble of life with young boys, and I recoiled in discomfort and pain, reproaching myself for my unmotherly reaction. I despised myself for my selfishness then and during our entire stay in France. I was ashamed of what I perceived to have been our inadequate gifts for our

The Episode

French hosts, which had in no way compensated for the warm hospitality we had been shown. I was also dreading the reaction of the three friends in Dublin who had been so supportive of me and the children since John's death. *If they haven't tired of me already, they certainly will now*, I thought as I imagined their dismay on realizing that not only had the holiday in France *not* brought an improvement, but I was further away than ever from my pre-bereavement self.

The day after our flight back to Ireland, I returned to my local medical centre, accompanied by R. This time I was met by the elderly gentleman doctor of the husband-and-wife team who ran the practice. '*Very anxious and worried about developing a dependence on anxiolytics*,' his notes of the visit state.

'There are some books I can recommend for anxiety,' he said after I had described my symptoms, and I scribbled down two titles, *Overcoming Anxiety* and *Self-help for Your Nerves*, neither of which I ever acquired because I was no longer able in my distress to focus on reading.

'I can change your medication,' the doctor added in a reaction that would be echoed each time I sought medical assistance for my physical suffering over the following weeks.

'A friend of mine said Paxil worked for her,' I suggested, attempting to be helpful.

'Well, we're not going to go with Paxil as there are risks associated with taking it. I'll give you a prescription for venlafaxine. It's an antidepressant but it also works for anxiety,' the doctor said, and he wrote up a prescription for 37.5mg daily, to increase after a week if necessary. He also told me to discontinue all the other drugs I had been taking intermittently since late June.

As R and I were leaving the premises, I asked her whether the GP had heard me talking about the burning. 'Yes, he definitely did,' she responded, but when I eventually read the clinical notes of the appointment, having requested them from the medical centre long after my recovery, I was unsurprised to see that they contained no reference at all to prickling or stinging or physical symptoms of any kind.

Over the following weekend, and for the first time since John's death, I felt hopeless about the future. I struggled to achieve anything beyond feeding my children and ensuring that they had clean clothes and enough sleep in the double bed where I lay awake at night jammed between them, my body on fire. I could cope with John's death, I told myself over and over, but I could not tolerate it if my health was broken and I was unable to create the new life I had glimpsed in rare moments of hopefulness over the previous months. I waited in vain for the venlafaxine to take effect. When I shared my belief that it wasn't working, I was advised repeatedly to seek psychiatric help – by my siblings over the phone, by the out-of-hours doctor who made a home visit on Saturday afternoon, and by the young female doctor in the Accident

The Episode

and Emergency department at St Vincent's Hospital who told me that the symptoms I was presenting with did not match any diagnostic category she had ever come across.

On Monday, 17 August, I returned in desperation to my local medical centre. This time it was my regular GP who saw me.

'Have you any thoughts of harming yourself?' she asked, her features set in an expression of deep concern.

'Well, if this burning doesn't stop, it's hard for me to see a future. All I've ever wanted since John died was to get better and start a new life with the boys, and now even that option doesn't seem to be available to me!'

'I'm going to increase your dose of venlafaxine to 75mg and refer you for an urgent mental health assessment,' the doctor said. In her letter to the community-based adult mental health service located a few miles from our home, she provided a brief overview of the four months since John's death. '*Today she feels she is not coping at all,*' the doctor also wrote, '*has some suicidal ideation and has thoughts of intent.*'

5

Crisis Assessment

On the morning of Wednesday, 19 August, I was seen at the local community mental health service by a member of the Crisis Assessment Team, while the boys stayed in my mother's home watching TV. During the assessment, which lasted approximately one hour, the nurse was attempting to evaluate my mental health, while I struggled to convey the severity of my physical symptoms to her.

'If anything you say to me today suggests a risk to yourself or anyone else, I will be obliged to report it,' I remember the nurse saying at the start of the assessment. 'Do you understand that?'

I was chilled by her words, certain that she was referring to my children and perhaps implying that I might be unfit to mind them. 'I understand,' I responded in a barely audible voice.

'Do you have thoughts of suicide?' she asked.

'No, I don't,' I answered truthfully. 'But I've had these pins and needles for over two weeks now, stinging pains and trembling in my hands. I think the medication has caused something to be messed up.'

The Episode

'Why did your GP's letter mention suicidal ideation?' the nurse persisted. 'What was it you said to her?'

'I was just saying that if this burning continues, I don't know how I can go on. I was trying to make her understand how bad it is. I'm desperately worried about it.'

'How about plans? Do you have any actual thoughts of ways to hurt yourself?'

'No, none. But I've felt physically sick. I can't rest or concentrate and I've no short-term memory. This has all happened since I started the medication. I'm not sure you understand how bad things are.'

'I *do* understand,' she stated repeatedly, but I remained sceptical because, while I returned again and again to my physical sensations, she seemed reluctant to discuss them with me.

'How's your sleep?' she asked, once again changing the subject.

'I'm not really sure. Not good, I guess.'

'What about last night?'

'About three hours, I think.'

'What about before that? What's your sleep pattern been like?'

'I can't remember. But that's the thing, my short-term memory is gone. And that's all since the medication was introduced. It's because of the stinging. I think my nerves are damaged and that I'll never recover. Can't you help me with that?' I had raised my voice and was almost beseeching her.

'Your symptoms can be treated,' she said, seeming to shut down the conversation, and I considered the word 'treated', which to my mind suggested something different from 'cured', the word I needed to hear.

At the end of the assessment, the nurse asked me to return the following day for a consultation with a psychiatrist. And two days later I was to present myself at the day centre operated by the mental health service. In her notes, she wrote that I presented *'as clearly agitated, unsettled, raised tone and rate of speech and very anxious'* and that my insight was limited: *'thinks ADT [antidepressant treatment] has caused permanent nerve damage and that she will not get better'*. The nurse also noted that following the assessment, she called the GP surgery *'to clarify what M said in context of "suicidal ideation" but [Dr] on holidays for remainder of week and notes do not elaborate on suicidal ideation'*.

The following afternoon, I met my first-ever psychiatrist, a younger female doctor with a pleasant smile and a nice dress sense, not too different from my own. Once again, the conversation, of which I have a clear memory, was captured in the medical notes of the appointment.

'How would you rate your mood out of ten?' 'Dr Gamma' began.

'Maybe two out of ten?' I responded, aware that no number could describe my unrelenting anguish and the self-loathing I was feeling at my inability to recover and at the obvious burden I represented to the unfortunate professionals forced to interact with me.

'How's your appetite?'

'I've no appetite. And I've lost a lot of weight over the last few months.'

'Do you have thoughts of suicide?'

'No, I don't. But I've had these horrible burning sensations in my hands and chest for almost three weeks now. Ever since I started the sertraline, in fact.'

'What about intentions? Any plans to kill yourself?'

'No, none at all,' I sighed. 'But I think there's a connection between the sertraline and the stinging. And I'm also worried about the sleeping tablets and the Xanax. That I'll become addicted.'

'Is there anything that you would identify as a protective factor that would stop you doing something to yourself?' she asked.

'Well, there's my children, of course. I want to get better, you know. I want to get back to the life I had before. But I don't know how to do that. And I feel bad for my children and also for my mother, who's been trying to help me.'

Dr Gamma then discussed my antidepressant medication with me. 'Will it work?' I asked, and she assured me that while the venlafaxine I had been taking since returning from France had yet to take effect, it was a very effective drug and should indeed work for me. She advised that she was maintaining the dose at 75mg, that she was introducing 0.5mg of

Crisis Assessment

clonazepam, a benzodiazepine with less risk of addiction than Xanax, to be taken twice daily, and that I was to start using the sleeping tablet zopiclone every night. '*M agreeable to same,*' Dr Gamma wrote in her notes of the appointment, though she also noted that I was '*reluctant to take meds*'.

As I drove home from my appointment with Dr Gamma, I received a phone call from the principal at my older son's primary school, where his younger brother was due to enrol in a week's time. (We had originally been unable to secure a place for him there, because the school was oversubscribed, but now it seemed that an effort was being made to accommodate us and relieve me of the burden of having to deal with two different schools.) When I recognized the principal's voice, I remember being immediately suspicious of her motivations.

'How has your summer been?' she asked.
'Good, yes, thanks.'
'Have you been away?'
'We've been to France.'
'And how are the children?'
'They're fine. We're all fine, thanks.'
'Have they been seeing their friends?' she probed further.
'Yes, they have, yes, of course,' I stammered while speculating whether someone had told her that I had not been managing to stick to my usual routine of organizing at least one playdate or one happy outing per day for my two sons. I

The Episode

was relieved when the call ended, so I could speed home to the children and wait for evening to come, when I could snuggle up between them and hope that the TV would distract me from the burning in my limbs and the threats emanating from the outside world.

My hold on reality had begun to loosen. It started with mistrust of authority figures who had a real or potential interest in my sons. According to clinical psychologist Lucy Johnstone, severe anxiety and paranoia 'often begin as responses to actual dangers', and I believe that the origins of the strange beliefs that would hold me captive over the following two months lay in the very real, distressing and perilous situation in which I found myself at this time. I was gripped by a terrifying – but I believe not unreasonable – fear that my physical suffering, and my inability to make myself heard, would soon make it impossible for me to care for my children and that they would be removed from me due to the lack of a family network to step in and offer support. On the evening of my crisis assessment, I shared my fears with my mother, who swore that she would never allow my children to be taken from me; but I was doubtful that she had the power to protect us.

My suspiciousness at this time also extended to the health professionals with whom I was starting to interact. I had some strange ideas about my medication and about the motivations of the people prescribing it. I had been asked to attend for a blood test before meeting Dr Gamma on the afternoon of 20 August. This raised two associations in my distressed mind, one hopeful and one fearful: I yearned for a physical cause to show up to explain the painful sensations in my body, but I also had a small suspicion that I was being tested for the presence of illicit drugs, especially when I visited the 'depot clinic' and saw that the other patients waiting there to be tested were pale and gaunt – *just like drug addicts*, I thought.

Sadly, no underlying physical explanation for my symptoms was discovered. Sadly too, my ideas about the torturing discomfort I was experiencing and the drugs I was ingesting were about to become much more bizarre, and increasingly alarming to the professionals with whom I soon started to share them.

6

Medication Madness

When I presented at the day centre for the first time on the morning of Friday, 21 August, I was met by a male nurse. He took careful notes of our conversation, including the following exchange which I remember very clearly:

'I need a physical examination,' I demanded before he could ask me any questions about my mood or appetite or sleep.

'I'm here to assess you for admission on to our programme,' the nurse replied.

'Can I see a doctor?' I persisted. 'Please? I feel nauseous and I have these awful stinging sensations on my forearms. They're there all the time.'

'It's not possible for me to arrange a physical examination for you today.'

'I think I know what's caused this, you know,' I exclaimed, and the nurse waited for me to continue.

'A few weeks ago when I was in France I took a sleeping pill a few times. Once or twice I split the tablet in two and took a half-dose. I'm really worried now that I shouldn't have done that. I think it's caused this to happen!'

I remember the nurse staring back at me in silent disbelief, the expression on his face revealing exactly what he thought. Perhaps he was right — perhaps I *was* already mad at this point — but I was still searching desperately for a rational explanation for my physical deterioration and mental decline.

That morning, I was allocated to Stream 1, described on the centre's website as 'a full time, rolling, open group, in which participants engage in a therapeutic mix of daily Group Therapy, Art Therapy, Drama and Mental Health Workshops'. The group sessions that morning were led by a young female nurse — I'll call her 'Brenda' — whose kind, sincere face would draw me into her confidence and prompt me to turn to her repeatedly in my distress over the following weeks. She wrote into the record that day that I *'engaged well, was observing and very actively listening to the group members, often nodding in agreement with what they were saying particularly during discussion around work, feeling overwhelmed by same and how to manage this'*. At the end of the session, Brenda met me briefly on my own.

'It was beneficial,' I said, when she asked me how I had found the group.

'Do you think you might try some of the suggestions to help your concentration at home over the weekend?'

'Yes, I'll try them,' I responded, and she gave me a number for an out-of-hours service should I need it.

*

The Episode

That weekend, I invested all my efforts into a desperate attempt to hide my symptoms from the children and to hold our routine together while my body was burning and I was crumbling under the strain of my physical and mental collapse. It is almost impossible to describe what it is like to run a home and to look after two young children when you have short-term memory loss and no ability to concentrate, and when more than anything else, you are craving rest. I would lurch from mealtime to mealtime, preparing food for the children, sometimes over-seasoning it because I couldn't remember whether I had added salt or not, and forgetting to eat myself, because I had no appetite and nobody to remind me to eat. My days were a frantic struggle to keep track of things I needed for survival – my keys, my wallet, my mobile phone and my multiple packs of medication. I would swallow a tablet as prescribed, and immediately forget whether I had taken it or not, or where I had put the stash of drugs. I was terrified of dropping a pill and would visualize my sons finding and swallowing it, almost as if I was reverting to an earlier phase of parenthood, when everything within reach of a crawling baby is a potential danger. To guard against this, I gathered up all the drugs into a paper bag that I attempted to keep with me at all times, carefully concealing the bag from the children when I went to bed with them at night.

Mostly what I would remember afterwards about the weekend of 22/23 August was an incident on the Sunday evening, when my friend R drove us to a nearby Tesco. There, for twenty terrifying minutes, I believed that I had lost my older son. I recall dragging his brother by the hand in a frantic search of the aisles and the busy car park outside the supermarket until I eventually found the boy in the frozen food section, where R had been minding him all along.

I also remember observing my two sons after we arrived home from Tesco, believing that their behaviour had deteriorated and that somehow it was my fault. Later that evening, I studied their sleeping faces next to me in bed, and a horrifying conviction took hold that they had swallowed my medication, and that their small, developing brains would never recover. I remember leaving the house in a state of extreme agitation, while the children and R slept upstairs. It was a humid night, and I wandered up to the top of our empty road, wearing pyjamas and a dressing gown and experiencing a small degree of soothing as the dark, silky air enveloped me. I stood watching the night bus hurtling past, wondering how it was possible for anyone to throw themselves under a moving vehicle at just the right moment, before returning home to a sleepless night filled with terror and remorse.

The following morning, I arrived early at the day centre, and asked to speak to nurse Brenda before the group therapy sessions began. I said nothing about the previous evening but told her that I was desperately worried about my medication because of my mental deterioration and the unrelenting,

The Episode

painful stinging under my skin. I wanted to be seen by a medical doctor and to have a physical examination, I insisted. Brenda's notes contain a detailed summary of what we discussed, including direct quotations from me:

'Can I speak to someone in charge, I don't think you can help me,' I remember demanding, after she had repeatedly turned down my request for a physical examination.

'You can talk to me. I can try and help you.'

'I think I'm being treated for an addiction!' I blurted out, remembering the gaunt faces of the other patients at the blood depot the previous week. 'You think I've been addicted in the past, it's obvious from what they've prescribed me. If I show you what they've prescribed you'll know why I think this.'

Brenda's normally placid features were fixed in a worried stare.

'I've been prescribed a highly addictive drug,' I continued, becoming more agitated and shifting my position on the chair. 'I want to know why.'

'Have you got your medication with you? Would you like to show it to me?' Brenda asked, so I took out the paper bag containing all the different packets of pills.

Brenda pointed at one of the packets and said: 'This is clonazepam. It's a benzodiazepine and it's good for anxiety. It's less addictive than Xanax and that's why you've been prescribed it. And this is venlafaxine, it's an antidepressant and it's not addictive at all.'

'I want to know what my diagnosis is,' I persisted, a trace of anger entering my voice.

'Well, you're here for further assessment and you're also being treated for depression.'

'I think it's more than that!' I exclaimed loudly. 'It's gone beyond that, I can't see depression having this bad an impact. Can I just have an honest assessment? Please?'

'Why do you think we're not being honest with you?'

'I think in my case you *do* know what's wrong and you're just not telling me! I'm feeling drugged, my functioning is getting worse, I'm foggy and my short-term memory is gone.' When Brenda didn't respond to this, I continued in an accusing tone: 'You think I'm cracked, don't you, because I'm not talking about my family?'

Afterwards, the nurse arranged for me to be seen by 'Dr Beta', a young male doctor with a pleasant manner and a kind face.

'I can feel the medication affecting my body,' I told him, having calmed myself down somewhat since my meeting with Brenda.

'These symptoms will settle in two to three weeks,' he attempted to reassure me. 'It's early days yet.'

'I suppose so,' I said, although I was not convinced. After all, I had *already* been waiting for two weeks for the symptoms to settle and there had been no change at all. Dr Beta wrote in his notes that I seemed to be suffering from the side-effects of my medication and that he had explained the purpose of the different drugs to me. I appeared to understand, he wrote, and to be *'happy enough with that'*.

Away from the day centre, I was struggling to hold our lives together while obsessing over the events of Sunday evening. My three close friends had found a nanny for me, who was a trained teacher and charged a steep fee for a full-time, live-out position. Apart from her, my mother, the children and my three friends, I tried to cut everyone else out of my life because I lacked the social skills required to manage appointments and make small talk with people outside my innermost sphere. When other friends contacted me, wanting to meet up, I would fend them off as best I could. 'Send me a text to remind me,' I would say if I was forced to make an arrangement, and then I would forget or attempt to postpone or cancel.

There were colleagues and acquaintances who hadn't seen me since the funeral, or even before, like my former PhD supervisor who had learned belatedly about our loss and wanted to offer condolences in person. I remember a stiff walk with her around our local park. I knew she was trying to connect with me, but I was unable to smile or make conversation. 'We didn't have enough time together,' I told her of John, silently willing her to go away so I could close the door on the outside world and return home to my children, where the downward trajectory would continue as I channelled my dwindling energies into looking after them, forgetting to wash myself or to change my clothes, and barely surviving on little or no food and on only a couple of hours' sleep every night.

During every waking moment, I searched deep to recall what had happened on Sunday evening. The children had suffered irreversible harm, of that I was certain; they had swallowed my medication and it was my fault, of these things I was equally sure. Now they were changed – less sharp, more unhappy, more prone to bad behaviour and bad language. But *how* had it happened? Perhaps I had dropped a tablet somewhere in the house and they had picked it up and ingested it? Or maybe I'd left the paper bag of drugs lying around –carelessly and unforgivably – and they'd found it? I relived every moment of the supermarket visit, remembering the meal I had cooked for all of us just beforehand. Maybe the medication had fallen from my bag into the pot of food bubbling on top of the cooker? But why would I have been holding the bag over the food while cooking? And surely my friend R, who had also been there, would have noticed? The more I rummaged for answers, the more it seemed that there could only be one explanation: I must have added the medication to the food intentionally. As the different scenarios whirled around in my head on a never-ending loop, I was tormented by an image of my evil self standing over the cooker on Sunday evening, pouring pills into the simmering food with the depraved intention of causing harm.

I thought I might test my belief on R, who had been staying most nights since I started attending the day centre – apart from when my mother was available to be with us. I recognized that R was worried about me and the children, and she seemed increasingly burdened by the need to spend so much time with us despite holding down a full-time job and having a household of her own to run.

'I know this is hard for you,' I began one evening during the week of 24 August. 'You're going to end up hating me.'

'Don't be silly!' R teased me.

'Honestly, you will. When I tell you what I've done.'

'Go on then, try me,' she said, still smiling.

'Well,' I hesitated, 'remember the meal we had on Sunday evening? Did you notice anything strange about it?'

'On Sunday? Anything *strange*?'

'Have you been feeling different? Since you ate it?'

'*Different?*'

I lowered my voice to make sure the children couldn't hear: 'I think there might have been medication in that food. It might have affected you.'

'Don't be ridiculous!' R snapped back at me.

I could see the alarm in her eyes and thought it best to let the subject drop. I knew that my words could be relayed back to the mental health professionals, who were in frequent communication with my three close friends because I had given the service my consent to contact them.

Meanwhile, I was continuing to present for therapy sessions every day from 11 a.m. to 3 p.m. While there, I engaged in a desperate struggle to create an impression of normality, while ruminating over what I believed had happened to my children on Sunday evening. I sat through the group therapies with my scorching legs coiled tightly around each other, and a bottomless reservoir of fear and dread lodged deep in the pit of my stomach. Brenda noted that I had been '*very vague about the weekend*' when I talked to her on Monday. But as the week wore on, I felt an irresistible urge to reveal to the nurse with the kind eyes and the sincere, open face what had happened, or what I *believed* had happened, on the evening of the supermarket visit.

'I've had some unusual behaviour,' I blurted out to her on Wednesday, 26 August after asking to speak to her in private. 'I left my house on Sunday night, I walked around and then I returned home.'

'*Was vague about this,*' Brenda wrote in her notes, which once again provide a detailed account of my jumbled narrative – which now extended to my children and was therefore guaranteed to alarm anyone who heard it.

'Why did you leave your house?' Brenda asked me.

'I was foggy and my short-term memory is gone.'

Brenda waited for me to elaborate.

'See, you'll have to report this,' I continued, becoming agitated, 'but my friend was staying with us, so the children weren't left alone.'

'What will I have to report?'

'I lost a tablet on Sunday evening and the children picked

it up and swallowed it,' I said, offering what seemed like the least self-incriminating narrative of all the different scenarios that were swirling round my head. 'There's a change in their behaviour, the older one is sick, their short-term memory has been affected,' I added.

Brenda looked at me wordlessly, her eyes wide with concern.

'If I did this, this would be the end for me. Could you assess the boys?' I pleaded with her.

'What tablet do you think you lost?'

'Clonazepam,' I responded. I had been in a heightened state of alarm over this class of drug ever since my GP had warned me about the addictive potential of Xanax in early July.

'How about you show me the box? So how many of these have you taken since Thursday?'

'Six, I think.'

'This is a pack of fourteen and there are eight left, so it doesn't look to me like you've lost any.'

'Well, I'm pretty sure there were more than fourteen in that pack to begin with. Anyway, I don't think these are clonazepam at all! I think they're something for addiction. The boys were tripping the other night!'

I remember the nurse's worried expression as I tried to persuade her of my guilt. She wrote in her notes that I held all my beliefs *with great conviction*. It might be more accurate to say that the beliefs held *me* in their steely grip, and that I was unable to shake them off or disprove them to myself because it was *my* cognition that was impaired, rather than that of my children. The nurse also wrote that I '*looked visibly anxious and remorseful*'; that I was '*appropriate*' in my emotional responses; that I had been keen to open up to her in order '*to do the right thing*' for my children; that my '*beliefs were in keeping with delusional thoughts*'; and that '*there were no immediate child welfare issues evident*'.

Following my conversation with Brenda, I was asked to return to the tall Victorian building that housed the mental health facility where my crisis assessment had taken place one week previously. I remember being met there by two psychiatrists, one male and one female, who inspected me with unsmiling faces as I entered the consultation room.

'Do you know why you're here?' the male psychiatrist asked.

'It's about my boys,' I answered.

'What's wrong with your boys?'

'Nothing,' I whispered, before sketching out the visit to the supermarket and my walk from the house on Sunday night.

'Somebody was looking after them when I left,' I added, 'in case you're concerned about that.'

'Anything else about your boys?'

'I think I might have dropped clonazepam into their food,' I said in a hushed voice.

'Well, we want you to take a new medication. An antipsychotic.' They explained briefly what antipsychotics are for, handing me an information leaflet about olanzapine, while I reflected on the word 'psychotic' and wondered whether it meant the same thing as 'psychopathic', with its connotations of unpredictability and violence.

'I'm not psychotic, you know,' I told them.

'Well, we still think you need to take this medication,' the male doctor continued as he wrote a prescription for a week's supply of 5mg of olanzapine to be taken nightly, telling me to have it filled on my way home and to take the first tablet before I went to bed.

'How long do I have to take it for?' I asked, fearful at the prospect of another drug and a label that I didn't believe applied to me.

'It doesn't matter how long, whether it's for one month or for three years. What matters is that you get better. You need to do this for yourself, and most of all, you need to do it for your children.'

I took the information leaflet and the prescription home with me, waiting before I got it filled, just as I had hesitated when the young locum had prescribed sertraline at my local medical centre some weeks previously.

After another tormented night, I rang the day centre from my home and asked to speak to Brenda. Once again, she kept detailed notes of what I said to her:

'I need to talk to you,' I said. 'There's something else about the boys. I'm afraid if I tell you, they'll be taken away.'

'How did you get on with the doctors yesterday?' Brenda asked in an apparent attempt to ease me into the conversation.

'I got on fine, thanks.'

'And is your mother with you?'

'Yes, she's here now.'

'So, what is it you wanted to tell me?'

'Well, when we were out shopping the other night, the children had taken something, they were on some kind of drug or something,' I said. Then I hinted – albeit by denying it – that I myself might have been directly culpable: 'All I can say is, *I* didn't give them anything. I should have taken them to A & E, but I didn't. Since then, they're gone mental.'

'How have they "gone mental"?'

'My older boy, he isn't able to do a lot of stuff he was doing before, he used to do a lot of programming, you know, and now he's not able to program at all!'

Brenda noted that at this point she heard my son in the background saying, '*Yes I can*,' and that she then asked to speak to my mother, who confirmed that I had not yet had the prescription for olanzapine filled. It was agreed that my mother and I would go together to the day centre, where we were met by Brenda and Dr Gamma.

'I'm going to increase your prescription for olanzapine to 10mg and I want you to drop into the pharmacy on your way home,' Dr Gamma said, directing her words at both me and my mother.

The Episode

'I hear you have concerns about your children?' she continued, addressing me.

'Yes, well, they're behaving differently,' I mumbled.

'Differently?'

'They're not as sharp mentally as before,' I said, trying to avoid eye contact with my mother.

'OK. And why do you think that is?'

'Well, I'm afraid I might have dropped some clonazepam into their food,' I whispered.

'We think you need to be admitted to hospital,' Dr Gamma said gently, and she wrote in her notes that my mother and I were *'partially insightful but accepting of this'*. She also noted: *'Fully delusional about her children acting differently and not being as sharp mentally as before. Blames herself for this.'*

The following day, I was informed that a bed was available for me in a large psychiatric hospital. Even at the time, I was aware of the fear of Brenda and her colleagues that guilt over my imagined crime might cause me to 'do something' to myself – or, worse still, to my children – and that this was the reason for my admission to hospital. However, aggression and violence towards myself or others was never a feature of my mental collapse. Brenda had noted that I was 'angry' when I had spoken to her the previous Monday, but this was a very rare instance in my records from four months of contact with mental health services in 2015 when an adjective suggesting any kind of mental energy was used to describe me. Otherwise, the records from this time are full of words that capture much more accurately my actual mental state, like *'fearful'*, *'guarded'*, *'remorseful'* and *'reluctant'*. Aggression and violence may be a feature of mental breakdown for some people, but what I went through tallies much more closely with the experience of American novelist and essayist William Styron, who, in his compelling memoir of depression, *Darkness Visible*, describes the 'madness of depression' as 'the antithesis of violence'. Styron refers to 'the sloweddown responses, near paralysis, psychic energy throttled back close to zero'. 'It is a storm indeed,' he writes, 'but [it is] a storm of murk.'

Sometimes, when I tell people my story and arrive at this juncture, I am asked what else the professionals could possibly have done to help me at that time. 'Not a lot,' I usually answer, although they might have listened to me more closely when I first came into contact with them, complaining of a *physical* affliction. Perhaps they could have communicated more clearly that they believed me when I said that my physical symptoms were real and excruciating, regardless of whether these were side-effects of medication or a manifestation of anxiety. But it was a fast-moving and alarming situation, not just for me. Healthcare workers are not mind-readers, and they didn't know what it felt like to be inside my head and inside my body. I was living alone with two young children, and I was out of touch with reality. I had talked about not seeing a future for myself, I had wandered

The Episode

around my road in my pyjamas in the middle of the night, and I believed I was guilty of a terrible crime towards my sons. I needed to be taken out of the situation I was in. More than anything, I needed rest. I actually *wanted* to be hospitalized and, regardless of whether or not I had suicidal 'intent', or what the doctors call 'agency', i.e. the ability to *act* on such 'intent', my GP's referral letter and the words I spoke to nurse Brenda ensured that a bed in a psychiatric hospital was made available for me.

7

Asylum

I was first admitted to hospital on the evening of Friday, 28 August 2015. I was driven there by my friend R, who told me later that it was heartbreaking to be instrumental in separating me from the children just a few months after John's death. I felt extreme guilt at leaving my sons without their one surviving parent, and hopelessness about the possibility of recovery, but I also experienced some relief at the prospect of resting my burning body and my tortured mind, and of being able to surrender myself to the care of other people. My friends K and D had offered without hesitation to take the children into their comfortable home. I knew I would never be able to thank them enough for their kindness and generosity, but I took some reassurance from the fact that they would have the support of our full-time nanny while I was gone. At the same time, I tormented myself with the knowledge that I would miss my younger son's first day at his older brother's school and that, in any case, my children's potential for long-term happiness and success had been destroyed as a result of my depravity.

The Episode

I don't remember much about the intake process on the evening of 28 August, but I do recall being asked by a nurse shortly after arriving on the ward whether I felt 'safe'. Her question stopped me in my tracks. I wondered what she meant, and what answer was expected of me. Looking around and spotting some male patients, I told the nurse that I felt unsafe because I was on a mixed ward. This may also have been the nurse who mentioned 'two weeks' to me as the likely duration of my hospital stay; or perhaps that came from my mother. Either way, this was the timeframe that was fixed in my mind almost as soon as I entered the hospital, and I was determined for everyone's sake to be well enough for discharge by the end of the two-week period.

Various records were compiled that evening on the basis of an intake interview and information received from the day centre. An 'Admission Summary' notes that I was *'tearful during admission process and anxious re length of stay and being able to go home'*. I had *'voiced suicidal ideation'*, but there was *'no plan or intent'*. *'Regrets admitting same'*, the summary continues, *'unsure of being in hospital. Wants to be at home with sons.'* A 'Physical Assessment' describes *'dishevelled appearance, unclean fingernails, evidence of neglect of self-care'*, while the weight recorded shows that I had lost fifteen kilos, or two-and-a-half stone, since John's death just over four months previously. None of the documentation compiled that evening contains mention of my feelings of guilt, although 'Consultant Notes' from the next morning state: *'Believes her children are not performing cognitively as well as they should, blames herself for same.'*

I remember the general air of lethargy and isolation in the psychiatric hospital. The ward was characterized by the absence of any kind of stimulation other than wall-mounted TV screens and a crowded smoking area that I, as one of very few non-smokers, never entered.

My treatment consisted almost entirely of medication. Shortly after I was admitted, my daily dose of the antidepressant venlafaxine was doubled to 150mg, while the other two medications – the antipsychotic olanzapine, 10mg every night, and the anxiolytic clonazepam, 0.5mg twice daily – continued to be administered at the same levels as before. 'Meds' were dispensed two times a day, once after breakfast and once before bed, and medication compliance was monitored closely.

My days were spent lying on top of my bed, fully clothed, staring at the window, communicating with no one. As I lay there in frozen fear, facing away from the world, my arms wrapped tightly around my torso, the events of late August and what I was convinced had happened on the evening of the supermarket visit played over and over in my mind. I had no doubt that the children had been damaged by my medication and that I had caused this to happen. *If only I could have been hospitalized sooner*, I said to myself repeatedly, *then the boys could have been spared*. I rehearsed each of the possible

The Episode

scenarios in a desperate search for answers that were not forthcoming. I put arguments to myself for and against the likelihood that the boys had picked up a pill, or multiple pills. I remembered the pot simmering on top of the cooker on the evening of the supermarket visit and I weighed up all the conceivable ways in which tablets could have entered the food without anyone noticing or tasting anything different. The terrifying image of my crazed self standing over the cooker would insert itself into my thoughts, and I would force my brain to banish it and return – almost in hope – to the possibility that the boys had found and ingested my medication without any malevolent input from me. Then I would pray for sleep to rescue me from my agitation, before the thoughts would start churning again, filling me with self-loathing and dread.

My interactions with the doctors took place almost exclusively at brief team meetings. Twice a week I was invited into a room with several professionals present – my consultant; at least one other doctor; perhaps a nurse or two and/or a social worker. (Later on, during my second admission, others would crowd into the room too – trainee nurses or visiting doctors and other professionals from other hospitals, bringing the total to six, seven, and even eight on one occasion.) Presumably, team meetings are intended to bring benefits to the patient by uniting the different disciplines involved in his or her care. But I recall feeling anxious, vulnerable and exposed at team meetings, as if a spotlight were being shone on me and I was a peculiar exhibit under inspection, especially by the visiting medics, who tended to observe me with professional interest while refraining from making any comment on the proceedings.

I had been assigned a female psychiatrist, 'Dr Alpha', to whom I was introduced at my first team meeting on 1 September, at which Dr Gamma, Dr Beta and a staff nurse were also present. As part of this first meeting, Dr Alpha asked how my children were doing.

'They're not what they were,' I muttered as the four professionals inspected me and waited for me to continue.

'What do you mean?' one of the team asked.

'There's a change in them.'

'Why do you think there's a change?'

'I think they took my medication,' I mumbled, too terrified to provide further detail. 'The children are more hyperactive,' I added.

'Well, why don't you talk to the school and ask whether they've noticed a change?' someone from the team suggested, and I agreed that this might be a good idea.

The following day, the staff nurse who had attended the team meeting raised the issue of the school in conversation with me. But the idea of contacting the principal to ask whether the boys had changed filled me with trepidation. Sooner or later, I reasoned, the school would make contact with me, especially once it had come to light that my sons

The Episode

were no longer able to do simple arithmetic (as I believed) or to make friends or to read anything more than the most basic text. When I pictured their school careers stretching out into the future, I saw a path filled with disappointment and ostracization, and I knew with certainty that the finger of blame for their failure would eventually be pointed at me.

Over the following ten days, I was to attend three more team meetings at which I divulged nothing further about the true nature of my terrifying conviction, partly because I was unable to verbalize for the watching professionals what I believed had happened, and partly because the belief itself filled me with horror, mortification and shame. I was also afraid that expressing it again could mean a longer stay in hospital and more time away from my children, so it seemed safest to say nothing further about it. Records of the meetings state that I had '*no guilty feelings towards children's care currently*' (4 September); '*denied believing that she had disadvantaged* [the children] *in any way*' (10 September); and '*does not feel guilty about the children now or at least the intensity has waned*' (11 September).

I remember being asked at one of these meetings whether I still believed that I had 'poisoned' my sons. I shook my head in shock and embarrassment, recoiling from the word 'poison' – which I was hearing for the first time in relation to my delusional belief – and screaming silently that *that* was not what I had meant. The fact that there seemed to be no word in the English language to denote the true nature of my crime only drove home for me the magnitude of my wrongdoing. I perceived myself to be the first person in history to have committed a crime of this heinous nature, made doubly reprehensible because I, as a mother, had perpetrated it against my children. The fact, moreover, that I was finding it so difficult to convey the specifics of what had happened only persuaded me further of the unprecedented character of my crime.

Apart from team meetings, I was urged repeatedly to avail of one-to-one time with the nursing staff. But I found myself unable to divulge what was really troubling me to the different nurses who would come and go from one day to the next, as shifts changed from morning to night and one staff member was replaced by another, only to appear again what seemed like a few hours later. I felt a mixture of mortification and fear to the pit of my stomach at the prospect of anyone else discovering my guilty secret, and when nurses attempted to engage me in conversation, I was unable to interact in a meaningful manner.

'How are your boys?' was a typical question at this time, and I would wonder how this particular nurse knew that I had children, and that they were boys rather than girls.

'How was the visit?' a different nurse asked after my sons had been in to see me with our nanny and my mother, and I stared back blankly, trying to ascertain whether the question was a trap.

The Episode

Whereas it is clear to me now that everyone involved in a patient's care needs to be aware of all the relevant facts about the patient, at the time it bothered me greatly that while I was protecting my most private anxieties very carefully, every professional interacting with me seemed to know all sorts of details about me that I hadn't shared with them directly, including the exact nature of my disclosures to nurse Brenda at the day centre the week before my admission. I have always been a very private person, and this didn't change while I was ill. Only a few people ever get to know all the facets of the 'real' me. The more important I consider an issue to be, the more carefully I select who to share it with; but in the psychiatric hospital, every utterance I had made since first coming into contact with the mental health service in mid-August seemed to be common knowledge. (Of course, it was common knowledge because it was all written down in my 'EPR', the Electronic Patient Record compiled on every in- and outpatient using the comprehensive networked Mental Health Information System (MHIS) deployed across the service, and apparently accessible to everyone involved in my treatment.)

When I did talk to the nurses, it was usually to ask how long I needed to stay in hospital or to express concern around my childcare arrangements. The nurses kept careful records of these conversations and entered their notes into my EPR.

'How long will I have to stay here?' I asked one of them a few days after my admission.

'We can't say how long it will be at this point.'

'I need to be home for my children,' I tried again. 'It's only going to get more difficult to organize childcare the longer I'm in here.'

'That's understandable, but you need to focus on your own recovery for now.'

'I have to get back to work, too. Maybe if I hadn't told my GP how I was really feeling, I wouldn't be here now.'

'You do know it's important that you tell us what you're thinking and feeling?'

'What would happen if I was to discharge myself?' I enquired, remembering that the voluntary nature of my admission had been mentioned to me when I was first admitted.

'Then holding power would have to be initiated,' I was told, and it was explained to me what this meant. I understood very little of what the nurse was saying, but it all sounded entirely 'non-voluntary' to me. To this day, I'm not sure what she was attempting to convey to me. Perhaps it related to the involuntary admission and detention in hospital of severely ill mental health patients, a process that involves invoking the Mental Health Act and is informally referred to as 'sectioning', after the relevant section of the Act. My best guess is that this nurse was warning me that, should I attempt to leave the hospital without the consent of

The Episode

my treating team, I would be 'sectioned'. Hours later, the expression 'holding power' was still reverberating through my body.

As the days went by and I became more anxious to be discharged home to my children, I reported an improvement in my mood. 'It's four out of ten,' I would reply when asked, or 'five out of ten'. And in some respects, I *was* improving. For the first time since John's death, I was eating three full meals a day, and I was sleeping through the night thanks in large part, I would imagine, to the medication I was taking. There had also been a gradual easing of the burning under my skin, which had eventually cleared up completely. But I barely noticed, because that obsession had given way to the conviction that I had destroyed my children's lives. I was telling white lies to the medical staff enquiring about my well-being – not because I was being deliberately dishonest but because I *wanted* what I was saying to be true and I wanted to return home to my sons. I had been informed on 4 September that we could aim for a discharge date of one week later, and on 10 September I was reviewed again by Dr Alpha, who approved me for overnight leave. I spent the time with my children in our friends' house before returning to the hospital the next morning for a final team meeting and discharge home, with instructions to start attending the day centre again from the following Monday morning.

I remember not everyone was happy about my discharge.

Asylum

As she helped me to pack, one of the nurses grumbled about Dr Alpha – it was all too rushed, she complained, and the nursing staff had not been properly briefed. My friends K and D also suggested to me that I wasn't ready for discharge and that neither they nor I had been adequately prepared. But I was unable to share my true thoughts and feelings with them or to explain the mixture of mortification, fear, wishful thinking and lack of opportunity that had caused me to conceal the guilty secret of my hideous crime from the watching professionals over the previous two weeks. Unbeknown to anyone else, the intensity of my feelings of guilt had not waned at all, and I was just as convinced as I had been on admission to hospital that my children had suffered catastrophic and irreversible damage as a result of my deplorable actions. I was still gravely out of touch with reality, yet I was being discharged home to the same set of circumstances that had led to me being hospitalized two weeks previously.

8

Into the Abyss

After my discharge from hospital, everyone I knew was eager for me to be better and for my ordeal to be over. 'You're so much brighter,' my mother smiled. 'It's great to see you back to your old self,' my friend D beamed at me, and I went to great efforts to meet their smiles with a happy response. The day after my discharge was John's birthday – our first without him – and my middle brother flew over from the UK to be with us for the weekend. In what would later become a ritual that the children and I repeat every year on 12 September, we bought John's favourite cake and climbed the Sugar Loaf in North Wicklow, where I had taken him on his first visit to Ireland almost exactly fifteen years previously.

'How do you think the boys are doing?' I asked my brother carefully as we approached the summit of the Sugar Loaf, with its spectacular views of the Irish Sea, the Dublin and Wicklow mountains and, on a good day, the peaks of Snowdonia in John's beloved Wales.

'Fantastically,' he smiled back, and I felt a stab of remorse at the secret knowledge that their future lives would be anything but fantastic thanks to my depraved act of late August.

When I showed up at the day centre at 11 a.m. the following Monday morning, they seemed surprised to see me.

'I was told to come here,' I explained, adding that I had been discharged from hospital the previous Friday.

'Well, normally *we* would contact *you*,' came the response. 'But you're here now, so you may as well join in if you like. Are you happy to continue with the Stream 1 programme for the coming week?'

'Yes.'

'Anything you'd like to ask?'

'Well, I'm a bit worried about confidentiality,' I said.

'All group members are aware of the confidentiality agreement that is signed on entry to the programme,' I was told, and I was provided with a copy of the 'Group Rules Contract' to sign (for the first time, I believe).

'How are you feeling about your loss?' the nurse asked me in a rare reference to John at this time.

'I might do some more bereavement counselling,' I said, remembering the soothing hours I'd spent in Michael's therapy rooms before the summer, and wishing myself back to that time.

'And your medications? Do you feel they're working?'

'Yes.'

'So you'll continue to take them?'

The Episode

'Of course.'
'Any other concerns?'
'No.'
'Any fears for your safety?'
'No.'
'Any thoughts of self-harm?'
'No, none at all.'

That week, I slotted back into the programme as best I could. The composition of the group had changed, and there wasn't a single individual remaining who had been there before my admission to hospital two weeks previously. I was struck by how much more vocal and self-assured the participants seemed to be this time around. There were a number of young women in the group who were immaculately turned out, and they in particular would engage with the (mostly male) group leaders in high-spirited, almost flirtatious, debates of a kind that I would normally relish. But I sat and observed the discussions in silent envy of the eloquence of the other participants, lost in agonizing thoughts and berating myself for not joining in. Occasionally I would be called upon to make a contribution, and then I would try hard to say something that might be expected or welcomed by the other participants.

As the days of that first week post-discharge went by, my friends K and D started to drop by almost every evening to help put the boys to bed. They also resumed the custom that had started after John's death of having all three of us to stay over at their comfortable, welcoming house for one night a week at weekends. My friend R, who had stayed overnight so often before I was admitted to hospital, came by most weekdays around dinner time, and other friends also took to calling in again with small gifts for the children or food for us to share. I was desperate for the recovery that they and everyone else thought was already happening. Most of all, I wanted to be better for the children's sake; and, now that the new academic year was about to start, I also wanted to return to work and to start interacting with colleagues and students again. But all the time I was obsessing about my evil act and beating myself up over it. *How COULD you?* I asked myself over and over. *Those poor, innocent children that you and John loved so much. And look what you've done to them with your medication.* An unbearable feeling of fright was lodged deep inside my body, and I was filled with self-loathing, which only intensified as I chided myself over my inability to recover. *Maybe if I can sleep tonight, I will feel differently in the morning*, I told myself every day. Or: *If I could just lie down now for a few hours, things might start to improve.* But I could never rest because I needed to tend to the children, and to get myself to the day centre, and occasionally to give my mother a hand as she went about her busy life. And even when I did manage to grab a short time in bed, I got no respite at all from the endless churning of my thoughts, which filled me with hopelessness and despair.

The Episode

Towards the end of the week, the same nurse who had interviewed me on Monday noted that I had '*attended all sessions in Stream 1 this week*', and that I was presenting as much brighter in mood, albeit '*a little guarded at times*'. In fact, I was exhausted from the effort of presenting a brighter front to the world while engaged in a relentless and futile battle with my inner demons. After dropping the children off at school that Wednesday, I rang the day centre to say I wouldn't be there until the afternoon. I had spotted a rare opportunity for rest, and I spent an agitated morning lying awake in bed listening to the nanny clattering around the house. I was at a loss as to what to ask her to do while my children were at school and I was at the day centre. There was only so much food she could prepare, so I suggested she clear out the playroom, a big job that would require several days' work. I don't know whether it was the large spiders she discovered when moving pieces of furniture, or whether it was me and the blank expression on my face, but towards the end of my first week home from hospital, she informed me that she was returning immediately to her home country. There was an urgent family matter, she said. No, she wouldn't be returning to Ireland, probably ever, and no, she didn't require a reference.

On Friday, 18 September, I told the staff at the day centre that I needed to make new arrangements around childcare. It was agreed that from now on, instead of the full programme, I would attend for half-days. During the following week, I dragged myself every morning to the day centre, where I would sit passively through group sessions, my body rigid with fear. I remember art therapy as being particularly terrifying because of the expectation that we, the participants, would create an artefact of some kind by the end of the hour. I dreaded those weekly sessions, which would start with mindful breathing, before an invitation would be issued to use the art materials on display in front of us. I would stare in alarm at my blank sheet of paper, afraid that nothing at all would occur to me. I also recall sitting uncomprehendingly through a session of music therapy while the other participants engaged in lively debate about John Lennon's song 'Imagine'. Two years later, I would start to use songs as a powerful means of unravelling and connecting with the emotions generated by the events of 2015, but at the time music held no meaning for me whatsoever.

My inability to benefit from the rich and varied programme on offer at the day centre was a further source of remorse and guilt for me. I remember a new participant turning up in a catatonic state some time during my second or third week back at the centre. Her story, we learned, had to do with bereavement and grief, and it resonated with mine, although she was older than me and there were no young children involved. Within what seemed like a few short days, she had undergone a dramatic transformation, and her bright smiles and happy chatter reinforced my own

The Episode

feelings of worthlessness and despair. I hated myself for not being able to respond as she had.

As the second week post-discharge wore on, I found myself in a frantic struggle to hold my life and that of my children together while descending ever deeper into the abyss. All my dwindling energies were channelled into looking after them. I would try desperately to keep enough food in the house, but I was unable to compile a coherent shopping list. When I did find myself wandering around a supermarket, I would stare in alarm at the piece of paper clutched in my hand, noticing that some items had been written down multiple times, and feeling stunned by the challenge of finding anything at all among the crowded shelves and teeming aisles. Having lost the power of recall also meant that I had no means of testing the veracity of my delusional belief. *DID I medicate the children in August?* I would ask myself over and over. *HOW did I do it?* I wondered ceaselessly, digging for memories of the circumstances.

I was still managing to take the children swimming and to the nearby park, but otherwise it was all I could do to keep them fed, clean, and with adequate sleep. Meanwhile, I neglected everything about myself, from eating, to personal hygiene, to communicating with my workplace about my ongoing absence. I stopped showering and brushing my teeth and washing my hair, and I wore the same clothes day and night. I remember the children pulling me up on this once when we were going to bed, and hastily pulling on a nightdress while a hot rush of shame spread up through my body, across my face and into the roots of my hair.

Apart from that incident, I think I succeeded in my desperate efforts to conceal what was happening from the children. The only strange thing about me from that period that my sons would ever speak about later was my heightened vigilance and tendency to startle easily. 'Remember the time you panicked over the computer virus? And we didn't even have a virus,' they will sometimes still tease me, and I laugh it off. 'What about the time you thought we couldn't do computer programming any more?' they'll say. 'And you thought there was something wrong with us because we didn't know the days of the week?' To this day, they don't know that when I said those things, I was gripped by fear and looking for confirmation of a deterioration that was not, in reality, taking place.

Friday, 25 September was to have been my finishing date at the day centre, but the nursing manager wrote in his notes that he '*was unsure as to* [my] *overall state*' during the morning session.

'Is everything OK?' he asked me in group. All the other participants seemed to hold their breath in anticipation of me finally contributing more than my customary few, monosyllabic words.

'It's all fine,' I responded after a short delay.

The Episode

'Are you *sure*?' the nursing manager persisted.

'Well, there *is* something, but I can't discuss it here.'

Afterwards he asked me to stay behind and elaborate.

'It's my children,' I said finally, unable to hold back any longer. 'They're not doing the things I ask them to and they're struggling in school.'

'How do you know they're struggling in school? Do you have any evidence for that?'

'Not really,' I whispered.

'Why didn't you tell us about this before? You know you can ask for a one-to-one session if you don't want to discuss things in group?'

'Thank you,' I said, silently cursing my inability to open up to him. 'The day centre is very good,' I added because I wanted to show my appreciation, even though I knew it was candour rather than gratitude that the nursing manager was looking for.

'Well, you need to come back here on Monday morning,' he said, 'and you know you have the out-of-hours number should you need it.'

That weekend, I attempted in vain to fend off the torment of my thoughts, while searching around in desperation for someone to share them with. I did not become an entirely different person during my breakdown, but the specific content of my delusional belief made me furtive and fearful and unable to trust even the people who I knew were trying to help. I couldn't confide in my mother or my siblings, of that

Into the Abyss

I was certain, as I was terrified of them finding out the disgraceful truth. Not my friends either, of that I was equally sure: I was acutely aware that this was a deeply worrying time for the three friends who had been catapulted into my shattered inner sphere, and I didn't want to burden them further and cause them to despise me when they learned the shocking details of my wrongdoing.

When I returned to the day centre on the morning of Monday, 28 September, the nursing manager arranged to meet me with Brenda, the nurse I had chosen as the target of my disclosures before my admission to hospital a month previously. Unable to hold back any longer, I decided spontaneously to confess to her and asked to speak to her in private.

'I medicated my children back in August!' I blurted out as soon as we were alone. 'I did it on purpose. I put a large amount of medication into their food by accident. And now they've changed.'

'Really?' Brenda asked carefully, a look of shock distorting her normally pleasant features. 'How have they changed?'

'There's cognitive and behavioural changes in both of them. They're struggling in school with maths. My younger son, he doesn't know the days of the week or the seasons any more.'

'But how can you be sure this means they've changed? Has anyone else said they've changed?'

'No one sees them for long enough,' I said, raising my

voice and despairing of my inability to make myself believed by Brenda or anyone else. 'I wish you could just *see* them and assess them, then *you'd* see it too.'

'I think this is a symptom of your illness.'

'No, you should be telling a guard about this, you know. You can't take it lightly!'

'We may need to increase your medication,' Brenda said, her face set in an expression of deep concern.

'Please don't do that. I don't *want* to be prescribed more medication.'

The nurse tried a different tack: 'How was your time in hospital?'

'It was useful,' I said. 'I felt less tense.'

'How about these thoughts around medicating your children? Did you have them then?'

'They never went away. I just didn't talk about them. I don't like talking about them, you know.'

'Do you have any thoughts of harm now?' Brenda asked me.

'No,' I answered miserably and truthfully.

'*Strong delusional beliefs about her children,*' Brenda wrote in her notes. '*Holds these with full conviction, preoccupied ++ about them.* [. . .] *No thoughts of hurting her children but there is a risk of her deteriorating further.*' She also wrote that I had '*no insight* [. . .] *and will not agree to increase in medication*'.

'Please don't tell the couple who looked after my children about this,' I implored Brenda before the conversation came to an end. '*Withdrew consent to speak with K and D,*' the nurse wrote afterwards in an internal email. '*I will contact her friend R to update her and highlight deterioration.*'

Directly after meeting Brenda, I was sent to Dr Gamma for review.

'Have you thoughts of suicide?' she asked.

'No,' I responded.

'How about harming others and your kids in particular?'

'No, none at all!' I protested, upset to be asked these questions again.

'I may need to increase your antipsychotic medication.'

'I don't want you to do that,' I pleaded.

Dr Gamma noted that I was '*not agreeable to have medication increased*', but at the end of the review she gave me a new prescription for an additional 5mg of olanzapine, bringing the overall dose to 15mg daily.

Two days later, on Wednesday, 30 September, I was invited to a multidisciplinary team review with Dr Beta, social worker 'Emer' and nurse Brenda. I sat facing the three professionals with my arms tightly folded across my body throughout the review.

'Do you feel you're coping with your current situation?' I was asked.

'I'm coping OK at home,' I responded, 'although there are practical issues with organizing the boys for school, that kind of thing.'

The Episode

'How *are* the boys? How are they coming to terms with the death of their father?'

'I think they're acting differently,' I said, averting my gaze. After a short pause, I added in a low voice: 'It's my fault and it's eating me up.'

'But do you remember a specific event where something happened with your medication?'

'No, but I know it happened and the boys will be permanently affected,' I said, convinced that what I was saying was true, and both wanting and not wanting to be believed.

'You have the option of returning to hospital if you think that might be helpful,' Dr Beta suggested. 'We could meet your friends to explain the current situation to them.'

'Thank you,' I said, 'I'll consider it.' But I no longer felt able to ask the three friends who had been so heavily involved in my life over the previous few months to attend a meeting with my medical team, let alone to ask them to mind my children again so as to enable me to return to hospital.

'There's also Barnardo's Child Bereavement Service and Tusla Family Support Service,' Emer added.

'Thanks, I'll consider those too,' I responded, certain that the first service would be of benefit, but unsure what the second might involve.

By the start of October, I was close to physical and mental collapse. My three friends had swung into action again to help me find a new childminder. 'P' was a quiet, well-educated young woman with a kind, intelligent face who had arrived in Ireland some weeks previously and was enrolled in an English-language course that ran in the mornings nearby. The interview took place in a café in Dun Laoghaire and my friend R accompanied me. She put all the right questions to P, while I rebuked myself silently for not knowing what to ask a stranger who, after all, would be looking after *my* children in *my* house. It was agreed that P would walk home with the boys after school each day and spend the afternoons in our house, and I hoped that my sons would adjust to yet another change at a time when there had already been so much disruption in their lives.

A second childminder with availability in the mornings had also been recommended to me, but I was unable to think of how she might help. After the nanny's hasty departure for reasons possibly related to the tasks I had assigned her, I was reluctant to suggest that the new childminder tackle the dirty dishes that would pile up by the kitchen sink every evening following P's departure. Because she had her own car, I gave this second minder the job of driving my sons to school. Every morning, she would pick them up at the agreed time, enabling me to spend the hour beforehand preparing lunchboxes for the boys and getting them dressed and fed, avoiding the need to dress and wash myself in preparation for dropping them at the school gates, where I was bound to be seen by people I knew. I was aware of the absurdity of paying a childminder for a full hour's work to

The Episode

do a ten-minute school run, and my inability to manage the two minders and make good use of their time only added to my overall sense of miserable failure.

Once the children left each morning, I would try to rest a little before summoning all my energy to drive the five miles to the day centre. *Just half an hour*, I would say to myself as I set the alarm on my mobile phone. On the morning of Tuesday, 6 October, I was unable to rouse myself for the 11 a.m. start. I managed to ring the day centre to let them know and was persuaded to attend for an afternoon consultation with the kind young psychiatrist Dr Beta. I remember him sharing some personal details with me by way of establishing a human rapport and easing me into the conversation:

'My father died when I was a young boy,' he said. 'This is what prompted me to become interested in medicine and to eventually choose psychiatry as a specialism.'

I smiled back at him, thinking that it wasn't difficult to imagine Dr Beta as a young boy, the same age as my sons were now, but a boy with a much brighter future ahead of him than that which I believed lay in store for my children thanks to my wicked act.

'My mother did a fantastic job of raising us all,' Dr Beta continued, and I knew that he had said this for my benefit. But hearing about other mothers' achievements in circumstances that I was sure were no less challenging than mine only made me feel worse about my own struggles.

'What about your thoughts around "the harm done to the boys"? They seem much stronger this week than last.'

'They were always strong,' I answered miserably. 'I've had them all along, right through my time in hospital and ever since I came back to the day centre.'

'Do you understand why we're worried about you and your children?'

'Yes, I do understand that, but I would never do anything to hurt myself or the boys.'

'If you did have concerns in this area, you would tell us, wouldn't you? Or your friends and family?'

'I definitely would,' I promised truthfully.

If only I could have had more conversations of this kind before and after my re-admission to hospital, I might have been able to develop a relationship of trust with a member of my treating team and receive the help I needed.

As part of our conversation that day, Dr Beta also raised the issue of re-admission with me.

'If I was a single woman I would come in,' I said.

'*I asked M to reflect on this,*' Dr Beta wrote in his notes. '*In other words she was of the opinion that she required hospital admission but that it was the practical side of organization around the boys that was stopping her. She agreed.*'

9

Whether You Want It or Not

On Wednesday, 7 October, I received a scheduled home visit at 4 p.m. from Dr Beta and social worker Emer. I had been unable to attend the day centre that morning, as I had an appointment with the Department of Social Protection (DSP) in Dublin city centre, where I was issued with a Public Services Card, which, it had been communicated to me, I would need as the recipient of a widow's pension. I remember driving into the city while the children were at school and panicking when I came out of my appointment to realize that I had forgotten where the car was parked. I might never have found it had I not glimpsed it by chance in a side street near the DSP offices. I still carry the Public Services Card in my wallet, although I don't ever remember being asked for it in order to avail of any service, and the grainy black-and-white photo of my frightened face staring out at me always brings back to me the terror and helplessness of early October 2015.

The two professionals who came to my house that afternoon had requested that my mother should also be present.

Whether You Want It or Not

She was noted by Dr Beta in his record of the visit to be '*very well at 90 years of age, a charming and wonderful lady*'. He asked me if it was OK to speak freely in front her, and I nodded that yes, it was OK. Dr Beta told my mother that I still believed I had harmed my children and he asked her how she felt we were getting on. 'Very well,' she smiled without hesitation, and she went on to talk about the loving bond I shared with my two sons, and how the older boy had matured and mellowed and become more openly affectionate since his father's death. '*Bernadette was very caring and spoke affectionately to M about her concerns,*' Dr Beta wrote in his notes. '*Bernadette tried to reassure M that both the boys were fine. Yes they had lost their father suddenly but they were coping well and that M should not worry. M although able at times to take comfort from her mother's words still seemed perturbed.*'

The two professionals were firm, but patient, as they urged me to re-admit myself to hospital and I responded repeatedly that I had no one to mind my children. '*Discussed at great length with M and Bernie the logistics and practical side of M coming into hospital in a planned fashion,*' Dr Beta noted. '*M and her mother felt that M could stay at home with the boys and take her medication on a daily basis.*' As the visit drew to a close, Emer informed me that she was making a child-protection referral to Tusla, the Child and Family Agency. She said: 'Tusla is there to help families in need of support.'

She also said: 'I am making this referral whether you want it or not.'

The Episode

Emer explained that the agency would be conducting an assessment, and I nodded mutely to indicate that I understood. In truth, I had very little understanding of what Tusla's role would be, and the prospect of a child-protection assessment filled me with terror.

After the psychiatric team had left my house that evening, I insisted on driving my mother back to her home. Aged ninety, she was still a familiar figure on the local roads, striding out gracefully in a colourful dress, her trolley in tow and her still beautiful auburn hair pinned up in a distinctive and elegant bun. She had been a non-driver all her life and would have thought nothing of walking the mile home that evening, but I could see that she was tired. As we drove along the same route that John had followed the day he died, she thanked me for the lift.

'I'm so grateful to you for thinking of me and my needs when things are so difficult for you. I'm really very touched.'

'What did you make of the meeting?' I ventured from the driver's seat.

'I'm happy about it, love,' she answered, to my surprise. 'I could tell there was something wrong, and I'm happy you're going to get the care you need.'

But all I could think of were the social worker's chilling words: 'whether you want it or not'.

The following day, I returned to the day centre as usual. As well as attending group, I had an appointment with 'Dr

Upsilon', who, I had been told, was intending to conduct an interview with me. This formed part of an assessment for first-time psychosis, but I don't believe I was aware of the purpose at the time. I recall answering 'no' to all of Dr Upsilon's questions and telling him that the only thing that was wrong was what I had done to my children. Dr Upsilon noted that I *'met criteria of presence of psychotic syndrome'* and that his assessment of me would *'continue on the week following 20th October'*.

On Friday morning, the childminder collected the children to bring them to school and I went back to bed with the ever-present hope that if only I could rest, I might start to feel a little better. As I lay there, I agonized over everything that had gone wrong over the previous few days – the referral to Tusla, the palpable frustration of my friends, my ongoing failure to contact work and give them an update on my progress, the pressure to return to hospital, and the impossibility of leaving my children without anyone to mind them. *Just another half-hour*, I kept promising myself that morning, before I eventually switched off my mobile phone in the hope that sleep might come. I lay restless on my bed for the entire morning, tormenting myself over how I had let everyone down – John, the children, my mother, my brothers and sisters, my friends, my employers, and the professionals who, as I was aware, were doing their best to help me.

The Episode

As I prayed for sleep to rescue me, I could hear the house phone ringing downstairs. I tried to block out the sound in the almost certain knowledge that staff from the day centre were attempting to make contact with me. Eventually, at around 1 p.m., I went downstairs and picked up the phone. A senior social worker from the mental health service introduced herself and urged me to present myself at the day centre.

'I'm not in a position to go there,' I answered. 'I've to be at the house when the children come back.'

'Do you have someone to help you with the children?'

'A minder,' I responded, and the social worker noted that I *'sounded guarded on the phone, not willing to elaborate on supports available'*.

'Why didn't you come in this morning?' she asked.

'I was sick. I stayed in bed.'

'What about your concerns about your children?'

'I still have those thoughts,' I whispered, shocked to realize that yet another person – one I had never met – was asking me about my secret disclosures.

'The day centre has been trying to contact you all morning, you know.'

'OK, I'm sorry. I'll answer now if they phone again.'

Shortly afterwards, I received a call from a staff nurse at the day centre. He took careful notes of what I said to him, writing that, '*M appeared quite nihilistic in her thought processes.*'

'I've pressed self-destruct, I've caused this,' I told him. 'I've run my finances into the ground, I've cut all my ties with work.'

'You're not responsible for everything, you know,' he said. 'And you've done very well to attend here every day.'

'Thank you,' I whispered, unable to derive any reassurance from his words.

'What about the children, how are they?' he asked.

'Well, you know the thoughts I have? I've done them.'

'What do you mean you've "done them"?'

'The things I've told you,' I said, on the cusp of disclosing the details of my crime to this nurse, who was speaking kindly to me. But I lost my nerve and diverted into a list of the other worries that had been preoccupying me all morning: 'running my finances into the ground, cutting ties with work, not talking to anyone'.

I was still alone in the house when Dr Gamma and 'Sue', a nurse I had previously met in hospital, arrived. '*We first interviewed M on her own,*' the record states, '*and then her kids came back home with the child minder.*' I remember showing the two professionals into the sitting-room and spending the rest of the afternoon with them there, while the children stayed in the kitchen, first with P until she finished work, and then on their own, apart from when I would go in to check on them and fix them some food.

While we were in the sitting-room, Dr Gamma and nurse

The Episode

Sue put numerous questions to me. According to their notes, they asked me why I hadn't attended that morning (*'felt very low in herself and went back to bed'*). They also questioned me about sleep and appetite (*'slept only a couple of hours last few nights; poor appetite and evident loss of weight noticed even in the last two weeks; lack of energy and poor concentration'*). They noted that I had *'feelings of guilt ++'*, *'worries about financial ruin'*, and *'ideas of worthlessness'*. Furthermore: *'previously elicited delusion of having poisoned her kids with medications continues to be held with intensity'* and *'fulfils all criteria for severe depression with psychotic features'*.

Dr Gamma's notes refer to a period of *'almost four hours'* in my house after the children had arrived home. It is difficult for me now to account for the passage of so much time, but I remember the interminable standoff as the two professionals urged me to re-admit myself to hospital in tones that became increasingly heavy with irritation as time went by. I also recall feeling embarrassed afterwards to realize that during all the hours they spent in my house, I had not offered them so much as a cup of tea.

As for why two presumably very busy mental health workers would devote so much time to persuading a patient to return to hospital – when the Mental Health Act allows for involuntary admission provided certain conditions are met – I can only speculate. I remember nurse Sue saying: 'We can arrange for you to be brought in against your will, but we don't want to have to do that.' My best guess – and it is only a guess, albeit one that is based on a careful examination of my medical records – is that Dr Gamma and nurse Sue did not have the authority to 'section' me, because that authority rested with my consultant, Dr Alpha; and Dr Alpha was not of the opinion that I needed to be hospitalized at all. While I had not seen her since my discharge four weeks earlier, Dr Alpha was still the head of my treating team, and according to an entry made in my patient record on the morning of Friday, 9 October, *'the team's current recommendation is not hospital admission but ongoing close monitoring of M's mental state'*. This entry was made by the senior social worker who had talked to me over the phone at 1 p.m. Prior to this, she had spoken on the phone to Dr Beta, who advised her of the team's position. It appears that the plan for the weekend had been to offer me weekend support in the form of home visits and an out-of-hours number. However, staff at the day centre had been so alarmed by my unexplained absence and by the two telephone exchanges with me that lunchtime that they now believed I required urgent hospitalization. Based on everything I've read in my patient record, I believe that when Dr Gamma and nurse Sue came to my house on the afternoon of 9 October, it was with the sole mission of persuading me to re-admit myself to hospital as a voluntary patient. I also believe that they had no intention of leaving until I agreed – regardless of how long it took or how much I might object that I had no one to mind my children.

The two professionals spent a long time discussing with

The Episode

me the logistical challenges of returning to hospital. They went through every imaginable care solution for my sons. With each suggestion, I answered that I did not believe that the people in question – my three close friends, my mother, my brother, my other siblings and other friends – were in a position to look after my sons for an open-ended period of time. I recall becoming fatigued by the stalemate and by the persistent questioning and I also remember searching for ways of supplying the two professionals with what they seemed to be looking for. *At least if you can't do what they're asking you to do, you can tell them what they want to hear*, my shattered brain seemed to be saying to me.

'Do you have thoughts of harm?' they asked me at one stage.

'I might want to kill myself,' I volunteered through a fog of exhaustion.

'How would you do that?'

'With a gun,' I responded, even though I had never once, at any point in my life, then or before, ever considered any method of ending my life, least of all with a gun.

'Have you tried to acquire a gun?'

'No. Never.'

Eventually Sue asked me to take out my phone. She told me to call my friends K and D and arrange for them to mind my children so I could return to hospital. Her tone suggested that she would not take 'no' for an answer, so I dialled my friends' number and D answered. We chatted briefly about her children and mine, while the two professionals sat with eyes fixed on me and arms folded tightly across their chests. I searched in vain for words to reveal to D the reason for my call and ended it after a couple of minutes.

'You didn't tell her, did you?' nurse Sue said in an accusing voice once I'd hung up. 'Give me that phone and I'll call her back. You need to go now and pack a bag for hospital. Probably best to pack some bags for the children too. And tell them what's happening.'

I could hear Sue's voice on the phone while I made my way upstairs and stared helplessly at the piles of clothes heaped up on beds and jammed into drawers. I found some holdalls and was still gazing blankly at them when I heard Sue yelling up, 'What's taking you so long?' so I stuffed toothbrushes and a change of clothes and a few small items of underwear into the bags. Then I entered the kitchen and stood by the breakfast table, where the children were sitting over their colouring books.

'I have to go back to hospital,' I said quietly, directing the words at my older son.

'Again?' he asked, his face crumpling, and my heart breaking all over again. 'When will you be back?'

'I'm sorry, darling,' I answered, silently cursing the inadequacy of my words. Then I told the children that my car was parked at the top of the road and that I needed to move it. 'You can come with me if you like,' I said, hoping to distract them.

The Episode

'The children need to stay here,' came the shouted order from Sue, so I walked on my own to the top of the road.

When I re-entered the house, the two professionals were standing in the hallway waiting for me. 'We've talked to your brother in the UK,' Sue informed me. 'He's coming to Dublin tomorrow. And your friends are arriving here shortly. You need to say goodbye now to the boys.'

I did as the nurse instructed and, as I made my way out to Dr Gamma's car, I passed my friends K and D in the driveway. I found it impossible to make eye contact with them: I was ashamed of my failure and of the renewed imposition on them. 'We need to have your house keys and the childminder's number,' I remember K saying, so I stopped to give him what he required while keeping my gaze fixed firmly on the ground.

As Dr Gamma drove towards the hospital, I chatted nervously to her. She had asked me for directions, and now I was second-guessing myself.

'I think this might be the wrong way, I think there might be a quicker route,' I said.

'This way is fine.'

'I didn't take you this way deliberately,' I said a few minutes later.

'This is just as direct as any other route,' Dr Gamma responded.

'I never would have brought you the wrong way on purpose.'

'Don't worry about it. It's fine.'

'You're very sick,' she added gently, 'and now you're going to get the help you need.'

An 'Admission Summary' created that evening states that I presented as *'guarded'* during the admission process, and that I felt *'unhappy with having to come back to hospital'* and *'guilty'* at being away from my children. Reference is also made to *'blunted affect'*, *'poor eye contact'*, and *'low rate and tone of speech'*. I was *'amenable and superficially pleasant'*, it is noted, *'but reluctant to elaborate on answers to questions'*. I remember the admitting doctor yawning during the process, and I wondered was she tired or merely bored by me and my confessions of guilt.

First thing the next morning, I received a call from my mother. 'He's not coming today,' she told me, referring to my brother in the UK. 'He says he'll be here later in the week or next weekend.' She also told me that, rather than taking the children to his own home the previous evening as I had expected, K had stayed over in our house, and that, unsurprisingly, he was not in a position to continue staying there every night. 'You'll have to come home,' my mother said in a further call later that morning, 'there's no one to mind the children.' I sought out the staff nurse allocated to my care and told her that the people currently looking after my children were no longer available. 'I'll have to leave the hospital,' I said. 'I've no other option.'

The Episode

I was persuaded to stay, and throughout the afternoon the nurse gave me regular updates about conversations she was having with my family and friends regarding the care of the children. '*Continued to present as agitated and tense,*' she wrote in my record. The nurse also noted that while I took some reassurance from her words, this was '*generally short lived*', and that I was on my '*mobile phone a lot throughout the afternoon*'. I *was* on my phone a lot that afternoon, where I learned that my friends were prepared to supervise the children's care for one week, with the help of childminders and other friends of mine, but that they then expected my family to take over. My younger sister called me from the US asking whether I wanted a full-time carer or a roster of minders to support our mother. 'You have to tell us what you want,' she sobbed over the phone, but I was unable to give her clear instructions or to understand exactly what it was that was causing her to be so distressed.

That evening, I was informed by my nurse that my brother in the UK had spoken to her and said he was looking into the possibility of having two childminders look after the children in shifts, with my mother there as a familiar figure to the children. *How's that supposed to work?* I fretted, thinking that if I hadn't been discharged by the end of the week, my sons would be taken into care.

Out of the blue, the nurse asked me: 'What reason would you have had to medicate your children?'

'I don't know,' I responded in a whisper.

'Well, you must have had some reason,' she persisted.

'I think I felt if I was going down, I was going to bring them down with me,' I said, trying to appease her by providing a rationale. 'Not in a suicide way,' I added when I saw the shocked look on her face, 'but by being drugged.'

If I had the chance today, I would ask this nurse why she had felt the compulsion to ask me those particular questions about my delusion at that particular juncture, and how it was that she expected to receive a meaningful response from me. I had entered the most acute phase of my breakdown, a time when I found myself unable to disagree with anyone, least of all the psychiatric staff whom I did my best to tell what I believed they wanted to hear.

When I was re-admitted to hospital, what I needed most was to rest my tortured brain and my exhausted body after the trauma of the previous months. I needed someone to put their arms around me and my children (metaphorically, and preferably physically too), and to unburden me from the terrible weight of responsibility I was shouldering. Most of all I needed to be wrapped in kindness and given time to recover. But what I was to get instead was a system that medicalized my distress, perceived me through the prism of 'risk', and subjected me to a range of assessments that would end up inflicting further harm on me at a time when I was broken, vulnerable and alone.

10

The Matter of My (Non-)compliance

Of all the self-incriminating details I offered up to the psychiatric staff questioning me over the weekend of my re-admission in October 2015, by far the most damaging to me was what I said to Dr Gamma and nurse Sue about medication when they were in my house on the Friday afternoon.

I had been asked repeatedly over the previous weeks by staff at the day centre whether I was taking my medication as prescribed, and each time I answered that I was. I had been discharged in September with strict instructions to take 150mg of venlafaxine every morning and 10mg of olanzapine before bed, and, during the four weeks I spent at home before being re-hospitalized, I was hypervigilant about sticking to this regime. It is true that I had little faith in the medication, and that I was worried (not irrationally) about side-effects. I studied the small print on the boxes of pills I picked up weekly from my local pharmacy, and read that venlafaxine can cause drowsiness, dizziness, weakness and tiredness, while olanzapine can cause dizziness and weakness,

The Matter of My (Non-)compliance

along with restlessness, sleeplessness, and – ironically – depression. But I took the drugs as instructed, partly because I have always had a healthy respect for professional medical advice, but mostly because I was desperate to recover.

Now, while I was in the sitting-room of my house with Dr Gamma and nurse Sue, answering questions about sleep and appetite and thoughts of harm, I was asked again whether I had been taking my medication as prescribed.

'Mostly,' I answered truthfully.

The two professionals waited for me to elaborate.

'Well, I haven't always taken the extra olanzapine,' I admitted, referring to the extra 5mg prescribed by Dr Gamma on 28 September when I had told both her and nurse Brenda that I didn't want to be prescribed additional medication on top of what I was already taking.

'Also,' I expanded, 'I didn't take any olanzapine last night.' (This was either because I had forgotten or because I had hoped that not taking it would make me feel better; it didn't.) 'But that was the only time I've missed it,' I hurried to add, as I perceived the expressions on the faces of the two professionals change from scepticism to disbelief to anger. '*Poor compliance with medication*,' nurse Sue wrote in her notes of the afternoon visit, four words that would have far-reaching consequences for me.

One of the first steps Dr Alpha took on the morning of Monday, 12 October, after my first weekend back in hospital, was to engage me in a conversation about my compliance

The Episode

over the previous four weeks. The paragraph she wrote into my patient record is worth quoting from because it gives a comprehensive and accurate account of what actually happened in the weeks prior to my re-admission.

'M reported that she had been taking her venlafaxine XR every morning as prescribed. [. . .] she took the additional 5mg of olanzapine [. . .] for one week after her dose of this medication had been increased. [. . .] she self-discontinued the additional 5mg of olanzapine after the one week because she considered that the higher dose of olanzapine was making her groggy. She reported a reduction in grogginess when she reduced the dose of olanzapine back to 10mg per day. She reported that she had neglected to take her prescribed olanzapine on one occasion.'

Dr Alpha seemed happy enough with my response, and following the conversation she changed my medication, discontinuing the olanzapine *'in view of M's description of increased lethargy, reduced energy level and tiredness'*, and replacing it with a different antipsychotic, paliperidone, 6mg daily. The antidepressant venlafaxine was 'augmented' to 225mg and a second antidepressant, bupropion 150mg, added. I was also prescribed a sleeping tablet, zopiclone, 7.5mg every evening with provision for a further 7.5mg as required, along with 0.25mg of the benzodiazepine clonazepam up to two times a day.

Yet even after Dr Alpha had documented the extremely limited extent of my 'non-compliance', further entries by other staff into my patient record relating to the period prior

The Matter of My (Non-)compliance

to my re-admission referred to '*poor compliance with medications*', and a '*hx* [history] *of non-adherence to prescribed medication*'. The matter of my 'non-compliance' was also discussed with my close friends and with social workers from Tusla. It would eventually become clear to me that these people had been left with a significantly exaggerated sense of the extent to which I had deviated from my prescribed dosages. Never mind the weeks of ingesting a cocktail of antidepressants, anxiolytics, sleeping tablets and antipsychotics as prescribed. Never mind the regular visits to the local pharmacist to get prescriptions filled at not inconsiderable expense. Never mind the unrelenting and increasingly arduous task of forcing my shattered brain to be vigilant as to *when* to take the medication and *where* to store it. Once the 'non-compliant' label had been applied to me, it was impossible to shake off.

As for why the pills I was so diligently swallowing throughout my first period in hospital and the weeks following hadn't made me better, I'm not sure. What I do know is that it was only after I was re-hospitalized, and more medication was added to the mix, that I would finally begin to respond to treatment.

11

Do They Like Colouring or Do They Like Lego?

I spent my first week back in hospital in a state of alarm over what was likely to happen when Tusla became involved with my family. I had been told that the agency would be conducting an assessment, and I was convinced that my wickedness would be made known publicly and that my children would be taken into care. There was a huge television hanging on the wall outside the room I shared with another patient, and the volume seemed to be turned up fully from morning until night. Every time I heard the jingle announcing the news, I waited in terror for the newsreader to broadcast the details of my crime. The only question in my mind was whether this would be the first item of news or whether a longer feature would be held over until later in the programme. I lay in bed hour after hour, rigid with fright as the booming voice of the newsreader reverberated through my body. I knew with certainty that it was only a matter of time before everyone knew the truth, and I wondered what kind of future I and my children could possibly have afterwards.

Do They Like Colouring or Do They Like Lego?

On 13 October, social worker Emer visited me briefly at my bedside. She told me that Tusla had allocated a social worker to my case and that we'd be meeting her tomorrow.

I felt my stomach turn and nodded that I understood.

'My mother can't look after the two children on her own, you know.'

'Well, your friends are helping. They don't view organizing for the care of your children as a burden. They've stated that.'

'Yeah, OK,' I said, while thinking that 'organizing for' their care was different from actually minding my sons. I knew that a number of my friends had come forward to help, but it very much did seem to me from the vantage point of my hospital bed that it *was* a burden for those involved.

The following day, before introducing me to the Tusla social worker, Emer talked to me again on the ward. 'The option of a short-term foster placement may be considered for your children,' she said. 'This is often arranged where a parent requires hospitalization due to a physical or mental health illness.'

Please not foster care! I implored her silently while nodding to indicate that I understood.

'How about organizing a visit for the boys?' I asked. 'They haven't seen me since I disappeared from home last Friday.'

'Why don't you discuss this with your friends? And then we can all go together to the family room.'

I don't remember my response to this, but I can picture

The Episode

myself fretting over why 'we all' needed to go to the family room 'together', and wondering anxiously whether I was being prevented from seeing my children alone.

I first met the Tusla social worker assigned to my case – I'll call her 'Orlaith' – on the afternoon of Wednesday, 14 October. The experience filled me with a deep and visceral fear. The meeting began at 2.30 p.m. in the visiting room on the ward with three social workers in attendance – Emer, Orlaith and her Tusla colleague whose name I never caught – alongside me, a fearful, miserable, broken shell of a human being. Orlaith had a large, stony face and an accusing sulk that remained fixed for the duration of the meeting, while I sat with my arms and legs tightly closed throughout.

'Tusla is here to support the family in a plan for the boys' care,' Orlaith began. 'Do you have any questions about that?'

'No,' I whispered.

'We would like to visit the children at home this afternoon. Perhaps you could describe them so we have an idea what they might like to do during the visit.'

I struggled to find any words with which to describe my sons.

'Well, do they like colouring or do they like Lego?' Orlaith persisted.

'They like Lego,' I volunteered finally.

'We also need to contact the boys' school. Do we have your consent to do that?'

Do They Like Colouring or Do They Like Lego?

I nodded silently. Afterwards, Orlaith noted that while I '*appeared to agree to every suggestion*', it was '*unclear whether* [I] *was able to give informed consent*'. At the end of the meeting, she handed me an information leaflet about the Child and Family Agency with her phone number written on it, and she promised to call me once the home visit was over.

I returned to my room and was joined there shortly afterwards by Emer.

'How did you find that?' she asked.

'I don't know why I was so nervous,' I said, attempting a weak smile.

But even being questioned about how I had found the experience of meeting Tusla social workers drove home to me the gravity of my situation and reinforced my feelings of impending doom. Lying on my bed for the rest of the day, I agonized over what had been said. I pictured the social workers visiting my sons' school – to ask *what* exactly? – and meeting my children without me, and I waited hour upon hour for Orlaith to phone. I wanted to hear directly from her the true horror of what she had found when she met my boys, but when we finally spoke – it may have been the next day and it may have been me who initiated the contact – Orlaith told me that they were 'great' and 'a credit' to me. I was certain I could hear a 'but' in her voice, and I waited for her to expand, but she ended the conversation by informing me that she would be in touch again 'soon'.

*

The Episode

All through my first week back in hospital, I was asked over and over again about 'thoughts of harm' by nurses and doctors who weren't familiar to me but who seemed to know all about me. Their incessant questioning, combined with my knowledge that I was being assessed by Tusla, had the effect of reinforcing my belief in my own guilt and of gradually eroding the small reserves of resilience and assertiveness that I had left, in much the same way as vulnerable suspects can be ground down during police interrogations. When asked about future-directed thoughts of harm towards myself or anyone else, I stated repeatedly (and truthfully) that I had none. Occasionally I offered my interrogators some crumbs of what they seemed to be looking for. I had '*fleeting thoughts of suicide*', I had told a nurse on the evening of my re-admission, but when probed further about this, I '*denied having formed a plan and also denied any intent*'. Mostly I held my ground on this point even as the probing intensified – '*has no plans to act*', the doctor who interviewed me on re-admission noted, '*denies experiencing any thoughts of self harm at the moment*', a nurse recorded a few days later. Very occasionally, and especially when I was afraid, I offered a little more, like when I told the registrar on call over the weekend of 10/11 October that I had '*dark thoughts*' which I was unwilling to discuss, and also that I had slipped a large number of tablets into my children's food and that I had done this both '*accidentally*' and '*on purpose*'.

Do They Like Colouring or Do They Like Lego?

There were moments of lucidity too, especially when I talked to Dr Alpha. She terrified me more than almost anyone else, but at least she was a familiar face. Almost uniquely, too, she usually found something positive to write about me in her notes, noting that I was *'polite and pleasant'*, *'not restless or fidgeting'* and *'not hostile or irritable'*.

'I would never harm myself because of the impact on my children,' I told her on 12 October, according to the notes in my patient record.

'Have you ever experienced thoughts of wanting to harm your children?'

'Never. My children mean everything to me.'

'Why is it you think that they might have ingested your medication? How could that have happened?'

'I've no idea how,' I responded.

I spoke to Dr Alpha in a similar vein on the following day when she visited me again by my bedside.

'Did you ever deliberately give medication to your children or leave it unattended so your children would take it?' she asked.

'No, I would never do that. I want the best for my children.'

'How do you feel about them now?'

'I love them very much. They mean everything to me.'

'Is it possible that they didn't swallow your medication at all? That the way they're presenting has to do with the fact that they're grieving for their father?'

The Episode

'I suppose that is possible,' I agreed, although I was not persuaded.

I wish so much that the hospital staff, including and especially Dr Alpha, could have asked me about something else. Could I not have been invited to describe and dwell upon one occasion in my life, preferably before John ever entered it, when I had experienced a sense of joy (swimming in the Atlantic Ocean) or adventure (picking apples in Tasmania) or achievement (passing all my university finals in Germany with flying colours despite the language challenge)? The record of my crisis assessment in August shows that the only time I smiled during that entire interview was when I mentioned the six years I had spent in Germany in my twenties, and I believe that I would always have been open to topics of this kind.

I appreciate that the psychiatric staff, first at the day centre and later at the psychiatric hospital, felt compelled to keep asking me questions about 'harm', especially because they could be held accountable if something terrible happened. But at no time during my breakdown did I ever cross the threshold into aggression or violence towards myself or anyone else — either in terms of behaviour, or when it came to plans or intentions. I understand that the mental health professionals could not have known this with any degree of certainty, but there were problems associated with their persistent questioning of me in this respect, particularly given the nature of

Do They Like Colouring or Do They Like Lego?

my delusion. The more I was questioned about 'harm' and the more I struggled to answer, the greater my delusions of guilt became, and the closer I moved to the susceptible and suggestible state in which I would eventually find myself at the peak of my depressive episode, when I was prepared to confess to anything.

As the week wore on, each day brought fresh questions and new interrogators. Nurses came and went and asked me about paranoid and psychotic thoughts. I was interviewed twice that week by a 'Dr Omicron' as part of the ongoing assessment for first-time psychosis. She described my presentation in her notes as *'good eye contact, limited rapport, unforthcoming at times [. . .] did not elaborate on answers [. . .] flat affect, smiled briefly [. . .] tense'*.

'Do you ever feel hopeless or have thoughts of suicide?' Dr Omicron asked me.

'Maybe sometimes. Before I came into hospital. But I would never act on those thoughts because of my children.'

'Have you had earlier episodes of depression in your life?'

'Never.'

'What about the "baby blues"?'

'No, never. The only thing I ever experienced was loneliness when I was a teenager, maybe some low mood for a few days at a time.'

'Can you talk a bit more about this?'

'Not really, it was a long time ago. I was lonely in my early thirties too, just before I got to know John.'

The Episode

'What about paranoid thoughts?'

'Well, sometimes I think people are looking at me or talking about me. But that has to do with the way I am at the moment.'

By Friday, 16 October, exactly a week to the day after I had been re-admitted, I was in a state of intolerable anguish and mental turmoil. I was consumed by guilt – 'normal' guilt about leaving my children in the care of other people and abandoning them to the possibility of foster care, and pathological guilt about my supposed crime towards them. My brother still had not arrived from the UK, and I felt responsible for the mess I was unable to sort while trapped in hospital. I was in the dark about Tusla's assessment, about how long it would last, about what questions would be asked of whom, about what the children's school would be told about the nature of the investigation, and about the implications of the entire process for us as a family. Finally, I had no idea who would help my mother, who by now had moved into my house with the children but was ill-equipped to care for them on her own, even with the support of childminders.

12

Quarry

First thing on the morning of Friday, 16 October, I was called to a team meeting with Drs Alpha and Beta, social worker Emer, a male staff nurse, and nurse Sue, whom I had last seen in my house one week previously and whose presence filled me with a mixture of embarrassment and fear.

'How are you feeling?' I was asked by a member of the team.

'Slightly better,' I said, making a feeble attempt to sound upbeat.

'Could you rate your mood out of ten?'

'It's five out of ten,' I responded.

'How's your sleep?'

'Not particularly good. It takes me about an hour to get to sleep. Sometimes I nap during the day and I lie down a lot.'

'How about your appetite?'

'Well, I've been eating more since I came to hospital,' I responded, once again trying to present myself in a positive light, despite the fact that a separate entry in my patient

The Episode

record from this time noted that I had lost a further three kilos since my admission a week previously.

'Have you any thoughts of harming yourself or others?'

'No, I don't,' I said to the five pairs of eyes observing me.

'And how are your children?'

'Fine, I think. I haven't seen them, but I've been in touch by telephone. Also I've seen my mother and she tells me how they're getting on.'

'What would you like to do over the weekend?'

'I'd like to go home,' I ventured.

'Maybe you could do that and return to the hospital after the weekend,' Dr Alpha answered to my surprise, and I nodded my head eagerly.

I don't remember why Dr Alpha's suggestion was rejected by the rest of the team, but the record states that '*a plan was then formulated that the children could come and visit M in the hospital over the weekend*'. It was put to me that the visit could be arranged by Emer and that the nursing staff would also liaise in this matter with my brother, who was expected from the UK at the weekend. This was all noted in the record of the team meeting, which also states that my uncle was travelling up from the country in order to help my mother with the children over the following days.

In this record of the meeting, I was described as '*flat in affect*', but inside I was bubbling over with agitation. I believed that I knew why Dr Alpha's proposal had been rebuffed. Over the previous days an idea had taken shape in my mind that the children would be taken away by social services at the end of the week. I had a very clear picture of when and how that was going to happen: once school finished on Friday afternoon, they would be met at the gates by gardaí and social workers, plucked from the crowd and whisked away. Then the story of what I had done would be broken to a scandalized media and the wider world. This, I believed, was the reason why I was being prevented from visiting my home and was being fobbed off with talk of a weekend visit to the hospital: it was because my children would no longer be living in our home. I wouldn't be seeing them over the weekend – or possibly ever again.

As time inched inexorably forward that day, I noticed that the door to the ward was open, so I drifted out and made my way down to the front door of the hospital. Nobody was paying any attention to me in the mêlée of staff, visitors and patients at the hospital entrance. I exited the building and strolled through the grounds and out to the road. I stood by the roadside for some time. After the incessant harm-related questioning over the previous week, I was aware that if the hospital staff knew where I was at that very moment as I watched the cars and buses hurtling past, they would immediately think I was planning suicide. But my only thought in this respect was to wonder, once again, how anyone could master the seemingly impossible logistical challenge of throwing themselves under a speeding vehicle at exactly the

The Episode

right moment. Then I turned my mind to the question of how I could make my way to my house to check whether the children had returned home after school.

I took a bus to Dun Laoghaire, and from there I travelled by DART to Dalkey. When I left the station, I waited for a while on the bridge over the railway line, looking down at the tracks and at the oncoming trains bursting through the tunnel entrance. Again, I considered in vague terms how a person might scramble down the railway bank and hurl themselves in front of an oncoming train. Years later, I would read Arnold Thomas Fanning's powerful memoir *Mind on Fire*, in which he describes covering similar territory to me the day he made his way to end his life on the railway tracks somewhere between Dalkey and Killiney. He came much, much closer to acting on his thoughts, and actually managed to climb on to the tracks, where he stood rooted to the spot as a train tore past, so close he could see the driver's shocked expression and startled eyes staring back at him. But in my case, the practicalities of even getting close to the track were far beyond me and I lacked the drive to act on my thoughts.

I decided to take the long way home from the station, up Ardbrugh Road, along the footpaths through the disused quarry and over Killiney Hill. I had lots of time on my hands before the children were due home from school, and following that route meant I could keep away from the main roads and was unlikely to meet anyone I knew. The steep path through the brush was picturesque and soothing. The physical motion of climbing the steps to the top of the quarry in the mild October air eased my agitation and brought a small sense of well-being and relief. When I reached the top, from where I could see the two arms of Dun Laoghaire harbour stretching out to sea, I looked down over the precipice at the sheer rockface below and knew I could never throw myself over. I lay in the long, dry grass and thought about how much I loved my children and longed to be sharing a bed with them again. I cursed my careless words to the psychiatric staff and wished I could disentangle the web of confusion and misunderstandings I had spun.

After some time lying down, my tranquillity was interrupted by the ringing of my phone. I guessed it was the hospital, and I managed initially to ignore the insistent jingling and to distract myself by musing over how long it might take the police to trace my mobile phone to Dalkey quarry. But the number on the display was my mother's, and the thought of her distress compelled me to answer.

'Where are you?' she implored.

'I've been telling lies,' I responded, referring to my contradictory statements to the medical staff over the previous few weeks – and to the fact that I simultaneously disbelieved my own guilty utterances while being possessed of a fierce conviction that they were true.

'They told me you've left the hospital and they've been trying to contact you.'

The Episode

'I'll tell them when they call back,' I promised.

Soon afterwards the phone rang again. This time, it was the ward manager insisting sternly that I tell him my whereabouts – which I did. Then I took a call from Emer. I had started strolling slowly towards our house from the top of the hill, and the notes she entered into my patient record tally with my recollection of the conversation we had as I walked:

'I'm very worried about the boys,' I said.

'Why are you worried about your boys?'

'I'm afraid they're going to be taken away.'

'What makes you think they'll be taken away?'

'I'm afraid because of the childminders and the arrangements.'

'I spoke to Orlaith from Tusla yesterday and again today and this is not currently the plan.'

'Well, why did they contact the school, so?'

'That's just part of a routine assessment of the family's needs. Actually, the school spoke positively about their behaviour and about how they're doing academically.'

'OK,' I responded, unconvinced.

'Can you tell me where you are?' Emer asked after a short silence.

'I'm near the house, just walking back now.'

'Are the boys with you?'

'No, I'm not home yet.'

'Do you think it would be helpful for you to talk to Orlaith from Tusla?'

'Yes, yes it would.'

Immediately afterwards, I received a call from Orlaith, and she suggested that we meet. We discussed the possibility of me making my way to her offices, but I told her that I wanted to see the children first. 'I'm nearly back home anyway,' I said.

When I arrived at the house, it was empty, as I had feared it might be. It was past the time for the children to be home from school, so I lifted the phone and dialled the landline number of my friends K and D, who had minded my children back in September. The phone was answered by D.

'I'm looking for the boys. Are they with you?' I asked.

'Where are you?' D enquired.

'I'm at the house. At home.'

The line went dead, so I called back, and this time the phone was answered by my younger son.

'We're watching TV,' he squeaked in the baby voice he had adopted since John's death. 'We're having a snack. And P's here with us.'

I listened in disbelief as I tried to process his words. I almost asked who 'P' was before remembering the childminder I had employed myself some weeks previously. A wave of relief washed over me with the realization that if my son was talking to me from our friends' house, then he and his older brother must be safe.

Things moved swiftly after that. K arrived at my front door, visibly distressed, announcing that he would drive me back

The Episode

to hospital. 'I'm meeting Orlaith here and I can't leave,' I objected, but he told me that Orlaith and Emer would be waiting for me on the ward. As we were talking, two plain-clothes policemen appeared at the front door.

'Everything all right, sir?' they asked K, who was standing beside me as the two gardaí eyed me up and down.

'It's all under control,' he reassured them. 'I'm driving her back to the hospital now.'

Once they had departed, having spent just a few moments chatting to us, K suggested to me that they were medical staff. But I knew exactly who they were, not least because I could see their squad car parked at the top of the road. I'd also been expecting the guards to become involved ever since I'd lain in the long grass by the disused quarry, attempting to block out the jarring noise of my phone.

Just as K and I were about to leave, my mother showed up in the hallway accompanied by her brother – my uncle – who was ten years her junior, a sprightly, energetic eighty-year-old, carrying his overnight bag.

'I'm here to help Bernie with the children,' he said, giving me a gentle smile.

I remember responding with a casual turn of phrase that I regretted almost immediately: 'Thanks for helping me in my hour of need,' I said, and my uncle smiled back at me. Afterwards I worried that he might have found the phrase frivolous, and that I had not managed to convey to him just how grateful I actually was.

As we drove back towards the hospital, I begged K to take me to his house so I could see my children. I didn't expect him to agree, and part of me was also testing him to see whether he was under instructions to keep me from them. 'It might upset the boys to see you looking so ill,' he said, keeping his eyes firmly fixed on the road ahead.

He brought me to the ward and handed me over to the nursing staff. I was then accompanied to a meeting room where the ward manager was waiting for me along with Emer and Orlaith from Tusla.

'Why did you leave the hospital?' I was asked.

'I wanted to check that the children were OK. I was worried about my mother too. She's ninety and she's looking after them,' I mumbled, keeping my gaze averted from the professionals staring at me, their features hardened into expressions of exasperation and fatigue.

'Why did you feel you needed to check on them?'

'I was afraid that Tusla was going to put them into foster care.'

'I do not have the authority to place your children into foster care,' Orlaith replied frostily.

Once the meeting had finished, I was transferred to a high-security locked ward. My mobile phone was taken from me along with anything at all that I could conceivably

The Episode

use to self-harm. The male nurse who helped me pack for the transfer seemed surprised that I had so few belongings, and all he could find to remove from me were shoelaces and a tie from my bag.

A note entered later that evening on to my patient record, after I had spent a few hours in my new surroundings, stated that I had *'settled quickly'* and *'was observed to be calm and appropriate on the ward'*.

13

False Confession

When I awoke in the locked ward on the morning of 17 October 2015, I was filled with mortification. I cringed as I remembered all the people who had been inconvenienced (the nursing staff, the gardaí, Emer, Orlaith), irritated (Orlaith again, the ward manager) or distressed by my disappearance from the hospital the previous day (my mother, my uncle, my friends). I wondered who else knew about what had happened (my siblings? the children? their school?), and I flinched at the memory of my younger son's high-pitched voice over the phone. As I relived the moment when I was led back on to the ward, I wished the ground would open up and swallow me in my shame. More than anything, I wanted to stay in bed with the sheets pulled over my head, but I was forced up and out by nursing staff because there were pills to be swallowed and questions to be answered and a routine to be adhered to in the voluntary/involuntary nature of life on a locked psychiatric ward.

For most of the first few days following my transfer into the new ward, I was suffering from unbearable nausea. There was a vile smell that made me feel queasy, and I couldn't figure out if it was a cleaning agent or whether it was something internal to me, perhaps caused by my medication. The smell of food was intolerable, and I remember vomiting hard into the sink of the bathroom closest to my room on my first morning on the ward. I was terrified of causing further fuss, so I cleaned up thoroughly after myself before telling the staff nurse assigned to my care that I felt unwell. As I understand it, this was why I was seen by the consultant-on-call that day. The doctor wrote a short overview of my case into her notes, including that I had gone AWOL the previous day.

'What seems to be the matter?' the doctor asked.

'I've been sick. I think the medication is different and that it might be causing me to feel unwell.'

'It's more likely to be a stomach bug,' she replied, before changing the subject. 'Why did you leave the hospital yesterday?'

'I was concerned about my children and that's why I left,' I said as another wave of nausea hit me. 'I wanted to check that they were OK.'

'What made you so "concerned"?'

I forced my exhausted brain to focus on the question and managed to produce a clear and accurate answer: 'It was because of speaking to the Tusla social worker. I was afraid she wasn't happy with the care arrangements.'

'How's your mood now?'

'It's OK. Up and down.' I was searching for answers that might make me more likeable to the doctor questioning me.

'Any thoughts of killing yourself?'

'Well, sometimes I wish I was dead,' I said slowly.

'Any plans of actually committing suicide?'

'No, I've none,' I responded, almost apologetic.

'Do you feel safe on the ward?'

'Yes, I do.'

Describing my appearance, the consultant wrote that I appeared tired, '*not tearful*' and '*somewhat downcast*'. There is no mention in her notes of nausea or vomiting, maybe because I didn't volunteer that information or maybe because I had removed all trace of the incident by cleaning up after myself so carefully.

Almost as soon as I arrived on the new ward, I experienced a precipitous and frightening worsening of my psychiatric symptoms. I was petrified of drawing further attention to myself. I was beginning to grasp too that words were my enemy, so, as far as possible, I suffered in silence.

I remember staring out of the window that Saturday, 17 October, seeing the empty basketball court and the still, autumnal landscape below, and being wholly convinced that I was dead. At some stage during the previous night, I had departed this life and had entered a strange parallel dimension where time was suspended, and where I would never again feel joy or sadness or any of the normal human emotions.

The Episode

That day, not believing that any kind of moral code existed in the detached reality in which I found myself, I helped myself to my room-mate's food. While she was outside our shared room, I examined her possessions and guzzled a dark-chocolate-pecan bar and a bag of jellies I found there. I remember the sweet taste of the chocolate and wishing I had known about dark-chocolate-pecan bars while I was still alive. Weeks later, having come to my senses and having been moved to a different room on the ward, I would try to catch the pecan-bar owner's eye across the lunch table, but she would avoid my gaze. I was ashamed over what I had done and I wanted to apologize, but how could I explain to her that I had acted out of a belief that I was dead?

When my brother walked into the parallel realm I was inhabiting that Saturday afternoon, I reacted with incredulity. I stared at him in stunned silence as he told me that he had arrived from England that morning. He had already met Orlaith, he said, and the children, who were doing very well. He had also interviewed a number of candidate child-minders, and selected three who would be helping my mother on a rolling twenty-four-hour basis. He seemed exhausted and overwrought. As we sat together in my hospital room, he took out his copy of the Saturday *Irish Times* and started to explain the techniques used to compile and decipher cryptic crossword clues, as I stared on in silent incomprehension. When my mother came to visit that evening, I reacted in the same disbelieving way to her unexpected appearance, mutely incredulous that she could so easily transition between my own domain after 'death' and the world that everyone else was inhabiting.

As the day progressed, I started to inspect my room-mate more closely. She was a good deal younger than me, but as the hours went by, I began to believe that there was a skeletal old woman lying there. Every time I raised the curtain separating our two beds to check on her appearance, she had aged some more. Sometimes she had a visitor – her mother, I presumed – and they would talk incessantly. Even then, I would pull back the curtain and stare. Eventually I became too petrified to inspect the wasted limbs, protruding teeth, ashen skin and grey strands of hair on the cadaver laid out beside me.

On Sunday, 18 October, I tried to isolate myself completely by staying in bed. I wasn't just physically unable to get up; I was filled with terror at the thought of what I might find behind the curtain dividing the room in two. I remember the anguish of lying prone for hours on end, mentally going through the list of people I had annoyed and disappointed over the previous days. Trays of food were brought to my bedside, and remained untouched until they were removed again some hours later. When asked how I was feeling, I was noted by the staff nurse assigned to my care to be '*monosyllabic on interactions*', responding, '*I'm fine, yes, thanks.*' I recall needing badly to urinate but being unable to face my interrogators and the other patients, and so forcing myself to stay put until I could bear the excruciating discomfort no longer. I also recollect someone vacuuming outside the door of my room for what seemed like the entire morning. I experienced the noise of the vacuum cleaner clattering against the closed door as a painful physical jarring that vibrated throughout my aching body and penetrated my jumbled and frightened thoughts.

I don't know exactly when I was first asked whether I was hiding medication, or how many times the question was put to me before the morning of Sunday, 18 October. It must have been at least twice, because I knew to expect the question again. When the small plastic cone containing a collection of pills was delivered to my bed that morning, I set two of the pills aside and placed them inside the top of my bedside locker, where they would be within easy reach the next time the question was put to me.

Eventually I emerged from my room to use the toilet. While I was out in the corridor, I noticed a big red button on the wall by the ward entrance. I was certain that it was a prop in the fictitious scene in which I found myself and that, if I pressed it, nothing would happen. Sure enough, no sound rang out when I touched the red button, but when I tested my theory for a second and then a third time, I was approached by the ward manager and instructed to stop. It was noted in my patient record that I spent brief periods sitting in the communal area, but that I continued to *'self isolate'* in my room. The staff nurse assigned to my care observed '*a paranoid flavour*' about me. She wrote that I '*entered nurses' station and looked at CCTV screens*', and that I was also '*observed to smell a slice of cake before eating it*'. She noted furthermore that '*personal hygiene requires attention despite staff encouragement to shower and launder clothes*'. I attended the dining room for the evening meal, and '*ate a small amount of scampi and chips*'. '*Observed to smell same prior to eating it also,*' the notes state, in a description that would not, I believe, be out of place in a zookeeper's or experimental psychologist's observations about a caged and frightened animal.

Towards evening, the nurse assigned to my care approached my bed. '*Staff attempted again to link in with M this pm,*' she wrote at the start of a comprehensive entry into my patient record which captures the detail of our conversation:

'Are you feeling paranoid?' the nurse asked me.

'Yes,' I answered, after slowly coming around from the trance-like state I had been in all day.

'Who are you feeling paranoid about? Anyone on the ward here?'

Again, I hesitated before answering, trying to understand the question and to gather my thoughts through a haze of exhaustion. 'Yes, the staff and the other patients,' I volunteered.

'Why are you paranoid about them?'

'They're going to stab me in the back,' I said, becoming more alert and warming to the exchange.

The Episode

'With what? An implement?'

'Yes, with a weapon.' Then I added: 'I'm feeling paranoid about my medication too. I'm being poisoned by it.'

'Did you take your pills this morning?'

Remembering the two tablets I had hidden away in preparation for this very question, I said: 'I took some of them.'

'*Some* of them? Where are the rest of your pills?'

'They're in my locker,' I answered, pointing over to where I had placed them earlier in the day.

After the nurse had retrieved the pills, her questioning of me grew more intense and my responses more grotesque. 'Did you have thoughts of harm when you left the hospital on Friday?' she asked.

Images of speeding cars and hurtling trains and the sheer rockface of the quarry edge flashed in front of me. 'Yes!' I exclaimed. 'I wanted to jump off a cliff!'

'Would you do this alone or with someone else?'

'I'd take the kids with me. *That's* what I wanted to do last Friday! I went to the cliff but the gardaí stopped me. I was worried about the boys, that the childminder would harm them.'

I remember the nurse asking me halfway through our exchange to accompany her to a meeting room on the ward where we met the on-call registrar, a male psychiatrist, 'Dr Tau', to whom I repeated the same disclosures. I felt almost euphoric at the freedom of finally being able to say 'Yes!' in response to the professionals' incessant questioning, and to use *their* language and *their* categories as I spewed out my confessions. I recall putting on a silly, clipped voice, and almost tut-tutting as I piled self-incrimination upon self-incrimination, as if to provide a third-person commentary on the content of my utterances. 'Look how *bad* she is,' I seemed to be saying. 'Can you believe how *evil* this person is?'

'What would you do now if you left the hospital?' Dr Tau asked.

'I would get my children and throw them off the cliff. Then I would throw myself over!' I answered, almost triumphant in the knowledge that I was confirming the professionals' worst fears about me.

'Have you had other thoughts of harm over the past week?'

'Yes! I wanted to throw myself out the window in my bedroom.'

'Did you check how to do that?'

'Yes,' I lied again, 'I checked the windows!'

Dr Tau made notes about my physical appearance and my presentation during the interview. *'Poor self care,'* he wrote, *'dirty nails, looks poorly nourished, tired.' 'Engaging when prompted,'* he wrote further, *'but difficult rapport. Appeared flat and low though smiled at the end of the interview, and exchanged humour i.e., laughed when we asked if her mother had brought any potentially harmful substances and replied "grapes".'*

Why did I do it? Why did I say such appalling things – none of which was true and none of which I believed, even at the time, and all of which were guaranteed to make my situation so much worse? Because I thought I was living in a parallel realm and believed that what I was saying didn't matter in the real world inhabited by everyone else? Because I was close to collapse, having barely eaten during the preceding weeks? Because of the effects of the antipsychotic medication on my prefrontal cortex, the part of the brain responsible for executive functions? Because it seemed to me that the professionals, with their faces of mistrust and frustration, believed that I was guilty of *something*, and I myself thought I was guilty too? Because I had been asked the same questions over and over for two months and I couldn't fight them off any more? Because I wanted to be agreeable and to give the medical staff what they seemed to be looking for?

In a 2009 paper on the causes, consequences and implications of false confessions, Richard A. Leo, an American professor of law and psychology, wrote that 'the mentally ill are especially vulnerable either to giving false confessions or to misunderstanding the context of their confessions, thus making statements against their own best interests that an average criminal suspect would not make'. Leo also refers to a distinction between three different types of false confession – *voluntary* (offered in the absence of interrogation), *compliant* (given in response to coercion, stress or pressure) and *persuaded* (when interrogation tactics cause an innocent suspect to doubt his or her memory and to become temporarily persuaded that he or she has committed the crime in question).

False Confession

My previous confessions to having damaged my children in some ill-defined way were so-called 'voluntary' confessions. I believed fiercely in the truth of what I was saying, no one had elicited those statements from me, and, like most other confessions of this kind, they resulted from an underlying psychological disorder. But my confessions of 18 October and the days following were of an entirely different nature: they were 'compliant' confessions. Such confessions, Leo writes, 'are made knowingly: the suspect admits guilt with the knowledge that he is innocent and that what he says is false'. Even while I was gobbing them out, I almost marvelled at the ridiculousness of my disclosures, and I didn't believe a word of what I was saying.

'Compliant' false confessions of the kind I made on the evening of 18 October usually occur in situations involving coercion. A police suspect exposed to threats and promises might confess in the hope of leniency, or simply to bring an intolerably stressful and anxiety-provoking situation to an end. I'm not suggesting that the nurses and doctors who treated me in the psychiatric hospital subjected me to overt intimidation and force; they didn't, and they didn't need to, for me to experience the situation as coercive. Mental illness itself can make people more susceptible to pressure: 'coercion can take place much more easily', Leo writes, 'and in situations that a "normal" person might not find coercive'. I was certainly impaired by my illness, but I believe that even a healthy person would have been intimidated by the

The Episode

situation in which I found myself. I was being held in a locked ward (even if my status was officially 'voluntary'). I was being assessed by Tusla, and the assessment was happening 'whether I wanted it or not'. Most importantly of all, my husband, best friend and most loyal advocate was dead, and I was separated from my children and isolated from everyone else who loved and trusted me.

My false confession had a number of fantastical aspects to it. 'I went to the cliff but the gardaí stopped me,' I told the staff nurse on the evening of 18 October, even though my only interaction with the police had been when the plainclothes officers called to the house just before I left again for the hospital. 'I checked the windows,' I told Dr Tau, although I had done no such thing. His notes also state that while I was speaking to him, I began rubbing under my right eye, where he noticed *'a circular cut'*. Asked what it was and what I was doing, Dr Tau noted that I said *'this was a self-inflicted cut [. . .] done a couple of nights ago, with an "implement"'*, even though I had no such implement and had inflicted no such wound. The clearest indication of all that I was making things up came later that evening after I had returned to my room, when a male nurse approached my bed.

'Are you hiding a weapon?' he asked. (It was noted in my patient record that this question was put to me because I *'was acting suspicious'* when staff entered my room.)

'Yes, I am,' I responded in a daze.

False Confession

'Where is it? Where have you hidden it?' came the frantic response.

'It's under the duvet,' I replied, and just as the nurse began to search under the covers, I held out my empty hands and exclaimed: 'There it is!'

'What is that?' he asked, the expression on his face a mixture of fear and disbelief.

'It's a screwdriver,' I responded, although I knew that there was nothing at all in my hands.

I am quite sure that I would have confessed to whatever I believed the medical staff wanted me to admit to. I admitted to having 'plans' and 'intentions' to cause harm to myself and to my children, and I provided hard evidence of non-adherence to medication by squirrelling away two pills and presenting them to the nursing staff when requested to do so. In short, I pleaded guilty to everything that I had been repeatedly grilled about over the previous days, weeks and even months (along with the embellishments of the gardaí at the quarry edge, the hospital window and the screwdriver). I was like the eponymous subject of the Danish memoir *Dear Luise*, a psychiatric patient brought before a court in Denmark in June 1996 in a deeply psychotic state. Luise was charged with arson, having fallen asleep with a cigarette burning and setting fire to her hospital bedding. She pleaded guilty to arson, but she also confessed to lots of other things, like killing all her children (she didn't have any children) and selling drugs in the US (she had never been to the US at that

The Episode

point, nor had she ever had anything to do with illicit drugs). She kept on pleading guilty until she threw up on the courtroom floor. Her mother, Dorrit Christensen, wrote *Dear Luise* about her daughter's experiences as a mental health patient before Luise's death at the age of thirty-two. Christensen also wrote an article at the time about the humiliating legal process which led to a sentence of mandatory treatment, and had it published in a Danish magazine under the headline 'Well, at least we don't burn witches any more.'

14

Specialled

Following our conversation on the evening of 18 October, Dr Tau made three changes to my treatment plan in consultation with the consultant-on-call over the weekend. He increased my clonazepam dose to 0.5mg up to two times daily and switched my antipsychotic drug from paliperidone 6mg to risperidone 6mg, to be given as an 'orodispersible' (melt-in-the-mouth) tablet. Dr Tau also placed me on twenty-four-hour 1:1 'special' nursing observation, which meant that I was to be shadowed day and night by a member of the nursing staff, even when I went to the bathroom. I first noticed a nurse sitting at the end of my bed that evening and wondered why she was there. Her face was lit up by the e-reader screen she held in her hands as I drifted off to sleep, and I felt a twinge of envy at her ability to engage in an activity which was so out of reach for me now and from which I had derived so much pleasure in the past. '*No engagement with myself or peers,*' the nurse noted at the end of her shift. '*Pleasant when spoken to. No worries or concerns voiced overnight.*'

On the morning of Monday, 19 October, barely twelve

The Episode

hours after my disclosures the previous evening, I received a visit at my bedside from Dr Upsilon. He was there to resume the psychosis assessment begun in the day centre over a week previously and continued by Dr Omicron in her two interviews of me during the week of 12 October. Dr Upsilon pulled the assessment documentation from his bag and began to interview me, while my nurse looked on. I remember the terrible struggle of searching for the 'right' answers through the disorienting fog of confusion that was enveloping me, and becoming increasingly fatigued, and slower to respond. My priority after the calamitous events of the previous evening was to keep myself safe, and I recall trying hard to force my worn-out brain to monitor my answers in order to ensure that they were not only 'correct' but also consistent with one another and with what I had said in earlier questioning sessions in the hospital and the day centre.

Dr Upsilon noted that I '*was co-operative with the assessment*' and '*had a reasonably good rapport*' but was '*superficial*' in my responses. We completed the 'Calgary Depression Scale' and then, as my lethargy grew, we moved on to the 'Scale for the Assessment of Positive Symptoms' (SAPS), which divides the so-called 'positive' symptoms of psychosis into four sub-scales – hallucinations, delusions, bizarre behaviour and formal thought disorder. As we started on the first sub-scale of the SAPS assessment, I agonized slowly over each answer, compelling my drugged-up brain to guess what the expected response might be. (Of course, there *were* no 'expected' or 'right' answers: SAPS is a straightforward assessment instrument.) It seemed safer not to answer 'no' to each question, and so I started to answer in the affirmative and to flesh out my responses.

'Have you ever heard voices?' Dr Upsilon wanted to know.

'Yes,' I said wearily. (In truth I'd never had an auditory hallucination.)

'Whose voices?' the doctor asked.

'Voices from the grave. My father and my husband,' I volunteered through the murkiness that made Dr Upsilon seem very far away from me. 'But I try not to believe that these experiences are true.'

He then suggested that we postpone the assessment to another day, and I accepted gratefully. 'You seem tired,' he said. 'How about you take these sheets and have a read of them yourself when you're feeling better? I'll pick them up from you next week.' Dr Upsilon was still standing by my bedside as I lay back, closed my eyes and surrendered to the fatigue.

I don't know how many hours I was allowed to rest before Dr Alpha appeared by my bed. It was the first time I had seen her since the team meeting three days previously, just before I had gone AWOL, and she seemed irate. I remember cowering in shame and confusion at her accusing questions, while my 1:1 nurse observed us. I felt like a wayward

The Episode

schoolchild, fearing that the teacher's trust and approval can never be regained.

In my despairing attempts to provide clear answers to Dr Alpha's insistent questions, I offered a bewildering jumble of fact and fiction, of lucidity and obliqueness.

'Why did you leave the hospital?' Dr Alpha asked.

'It was a spur-of-the-moment decision,' I said, summoning up all my powers of concentration and managing to produce a lucid and truthful response. 'I went home hoping to meet up with my sons.'

'What did you do while you were at the quarry?' she probed further, and I felt the panic rising in me as I tried to remember what exactly it was that I had been doing there.

'I spent about thirty minutes looking into it thinking my sons might be better off if I was dead,' I lied, keeping my eyes fixed firmly on the bed in front of me.

'What made you think that?'

'I'm worried about the childcare arrangements and my ninety-year-old mother. I'm also concerned that there's no continuity with the different childminders. I'm afraid this will reduce the children's intelligence level further and make their behaviour even worse.'

'Reduce it "further"? What do you mean by that?'

'I've poisoned my children,' I blurted out finally, freely using the word 'poison', though I did not believe it to be a suitable descriptor for the crime of destroying my children's minds; rather, having heard others use it, I had come to recognize its metaphorical power. Remembering the vomiting incident two days previously, I also added, 'I think I'm being poisoned by my medication.'

'Have you any thoughts or plans to harm your children now?'

'No, none,' I responded truthfully.

Dr Alpha noted my non-verbal behaviour during the meeting as '*intermittent eye contact* [. . .] *looking downwards for the remainder of the time at her bed on which she was sitting*'. Even then, my consultant found something positive to write about me: '*clothes appeared clean* [. . .] *hygiene was adequate* [. . .] *speech was normal in volume and rate but was monotone.*' She put strange questions to me about '*thought insertion, thought withdrawal, thought echo and thought broadcasting*', all of which I denied, along with questions about '*hallucinations in all modalities*'.

'Do you hear voices?' Dr Alpha asked.

'No,' I responded accurately, while acutely aware of the presence of my nurse, who had also witnessed Dr Upsilon's interview earlier in the day, during which, as far as I could recall, I had said something different.

'If you ever leave the hospital again without permission, the Mental Health Act will be invoked and you will be detained against your will,' Dr Alpha cautioned me towards the end of our meeting. 'Do you understand that?'

I indicated mutely that I understood and mumbled truthfully, 'I won't ever do it again.'

I also plucked up the courage to ask about my children. 'When will I see them again?' I enquired.

The Episode

'Tusla is dealing with the child-protection issue of your sons,' Dr Alpha replied, and I retreated in dejection from the question of when my children would be permitted to visit me.

Shortly after my first weekend on the locked ward, I was moved without notice or explanation to a new bed in a different room. I never learned the reason, and there's no mention of a transfer in my patient record. I can only imagine that it must have been because my room-mate had complained about the madwoman in the bed next to hers.

Almost as soon as I had settled into my new surroundings with my new companion, a fog of dread and mortification descended over me. I was horrified at the words I had uttered, terrified of anyone else hearing about them, and incapable of comprehending what had driven me to say them. As I lay stretched out on my bed, I tried in vain to untangle for myself the web of confusion I had spun and I concluded that it was safer, and less exhausting, not to attempt to reveal anything further of any significance to anyone. Not to my mother, who was visiting every day, not to the nursing staff, not to my new room-mate who frightened me with her dark mumblings, and certainly not to my consultant psychiatrist, whose presence generated overwhelming feelings of panic, apprehension and dread in me.

Before I could clam up completely, Dr Alpha paid me another visit. It was Wednesday, 21 October, exactly six months to the day since John's death. I was painfully aware of the half-year anniversary and was gripped by shock and disbelief at what had befallen me and the children since the joyful occasion of my fiftieth birthday party just a few days before he died. Dr Alpha had an air of pique about her that day, and I remember how hard she was on me as she conducted her interview by my bed, with my 1:1 nurse for the day also in attendance. When she first arrived in my room, Dr Alpha found me *'lying in bed on* [. . .] *left side facing the wall with* [. . .] *eyes open'*. She noted that my hair was untidy, and that during our interaction, I was *'notably guarded and evasive'* and that I provided *'limited responses'* to her questions.

'I want to ask you about what you said to me two days ago in relation to the thoughts you experienced while you were absent without leave from hospital,' she began.

I *'notably grimaced'* on hearing this question, according to an entry Dr Alpha made in my patient record. I recall wanting to recant my false disclosures of the previous few days but being unable to start to explain to my consultant why I had made them. With two sets of eyes trained on me, all I could think of to say in relation to my thoughts while AWOL was: 'I can't remember saying this.' Dr Alpha made no comment in response, so I stammered: 'I can't recall experiencing such thoughts at all.'

My consultant then moved on to the topic of hallucinations and noted that I *'denied hallucinations in all modalities'*. I still have a clear recollection of the exchange that took place

The Episode

between us, the details of which are also captured in Dr Alpha's notes:

'Do you hear voices?' she asked, as my nurse looked on.

'No, never,' I responded truthfully.

'You told Dr Upsilon two days ago that you had been hearing voices but when I spoke to you that same day, you told me that you never heard voices. How do you explain the difference?'

I squirmed in discomfort at being pressed on this point and felt a deep sense of shame. I didn't know how to admit that I had been exhausted by Dr Upsilon's questions and that my statement to him had been false. 'I must have misunderstood the doctor's question,' I muttered to Dr Alpha instead.

'Well, what interpretation did you take from his question when he asked you whether or not you had been hearing voices?'

'I don't know,' I said, unable to come up with a better response while confronted with the disbelieving and peeved expression on Dr Alpha's face.

Before the end of the interview, Dr Alpha asked me to tell her why I believed I was in hospital.

'It's to get better,' I responded.

'Why do you think you need to "get better"?'

'My mood?'

'Can you explain to me why your friends – who have known your sons since they were born – have not noticed any changes in your children's behaviour or their intelligence?'

Specialled

I shook my head and replied, 'They don't know them like I do.'

'Have you ever asked either or both of your children whether they took your medication at any stage?'

'No, I haven't. I don't want to worry them about it.'

'What about the teardrop your nurse saw in the corner of one of your eyes this morning?' Dr Alpha asked suddenly, and I recoiled in disbelief at her bizarre question.

'I don't remember having a teardrop in my eye. I don't think that ever happened,' I responded.

After the developments of 18–21 October, I directed all my depleted energies at protecting myself from further questions and interrogations. As I sought safety, I adopted the same strategy as the abused children described in Judith Herman's *Trauma and Recovery*, who try to gain control of the situation they are in by 'being good'. Herman describes the efforts of such children to remain as inconspicuous as possible and to avoid attracting attention 'by freezing in place, crouching, rolling up in a ball, or keeping their face expressionless'. I remember the enormous effort it took to maintain my front to the nursing staff while seizing up with anxiety on the inside, just like the children Herman writes about who 'while in a constant state of autonomic hyperarousal [. . .] must also be quiet and immobile, avoiding any physical display of their inner agitation'.

I wasn't the only one to retreat. The interview on

The Episode

21 October was, I believe, the last time any psychiatrist in that hospital attempted to engage with me in a meaningful way about either the delusional belief that had afflicted me since late August, or about the entirely different (and false) disclosures that I had made in the days following my absence from the hospital in October. Over the following two months, as I regained my sanity under the watchful eyes of the hospital staff, I would be left on my own to deal with my pathological guilt and with the psychological consequences of having made a false and highly damaging confession. I would also be left to my own devices to cope with the very real consequences of my disclosures, some of which I was aware of straight away, while others only became apparent later. It is worthy of note too that had I really harboured homicidal thoughts towards my children, I would have been left without any therapeutic intervention to help me come to terms with the enormous guilt of having held such thoughts in the first place, not to mention the vital importance of addressing with me the provenance, severity and duration of such thoughts. There was no therapeutic agenda beyond medication, and the type of talk that the mental health professionals did engage in only made things worse for me.

15

Metamorphosis

When I was a student in West Germany in the 1980s, I studied the literature of Franz Kafka for my university finals. Kafka was a German-speaking Czech author who combined elements of realism and the surreal in his writing. One of his best-known works is *The Metamorphosis*, in which Gregor Samsa, a travelling salesman, awakens from anxious dreams to discover that he has been transformed overnight into 'a monstrous vermin'. Many different interpretations have been given to the transformation of Gregor Samsa. For instance, it has been seen as an expression of Gregor's estrangement from his birth family or as representing the alienation of modern man from his true self in the pursuit of money and material success. But it seems to me that it could also be interpreted as a particularly apt metaphor for the experience of awakening from an episode of psychosis to find yourself in a locked ward in a psychiatric hospital, under constant observation, and unable to communicate to anyone the truth of what has happened.

Unlike Gregor Samsa's transformation, my own transition

The Episode

back to 'normality' happened very gradually, over a period of several weeks. Even by the time Dr Alpha conducted her 'teardrop' interview with me on John's six-month anniversary and asked me whether I had ever tested my delusional belief with my friends or even directly with my children, I was starting to glimpse the possibility that it was unwarranted and ludicrous. Furthermore, almost as soon as I had made my false confession, I understood the seriousness of what I had said, and wanted to retract it. But I was terrified of making further mistakes, so I remained almost completely mute.

Very gradually, as I lay on my bed, my hold on reality started to shift from believing I was inhabiting a parallel world of pretence and delusion to comprehending that I had woken up to a brutal reality that was just as punitive and hardly less surreal, full of misunderstanding, loneliness and blame. For a number of weeks, I oscillated between the two realms on my trajectory back to sanity. Then, as my perceptions shifted, one set of anxieties and self-admonishments gave way to another; but while the anxiety triggered by my fixed delusion had been groundless and a product of my mental breakdown, the new fears that tormented me were anything but illusory. A visceral sense of impending doom had been my constant companion since early August. Apprehension and dread remained lodged deep inside my body, but now, the source of this intensely unpleasant physical sensation was changing from a vague and objectless anxiety to fear, or rather, *multiple* fears, the objects of which were specific, concrete, and very real: fear of losing my children; fear of the open-ended nature of my confinement; fear for my job (because I had not kept my employers sufficiently informed of the reasons for my absence); fear for my finances (my mother was spending €1,000 a week of my money on child-minders); and fear of the long-term effects of the heavy medication regime I was on.

I remember the extreme agitation in relation to my children that team meetings provoked in me at this time. On the morning of Friday, 23 October, I was seen on a ward round by a team of five staff – Drs Alpha and Beta, social worker Emer and two nurses. I '*appeared tired*' and '*came across as very low in mood*', my patient record states. It also contains detailed notes of the conversation and the exact words spoken by me and typed directly into my record at the meeting:

'Have you any thoughts of self-harm at the moment?' I was asked at the start.

'None,' I responded wearily.

'Any worries or concerns?'

'I worry about the boys and not being with them. I think I'll be here for ever.'

'Have you any other concerns or worries?' the team wanted to know.

'What about seeing the boys? When can I see them?'

'That is the remit of our social-work team,' Dr Alpha explained, and I nodded that I understood. 'Do you remember

The Episode

the thoughts you were having last Friday in relation to yourself and the boys?'

I was at a loss to know what answer to provide for the five pairs of eyes watching me, so I mumbled, 'No, I can't remember, I don't think I can recall them at the moment.'

'Is there anything else you would like to ask us now?'

'Yes,' I ventured again. 'What will the outcome of Tusla's assessment be? Will I ever be able to care for the boys myself again?'

'An inter-agency meeting will be convened shortly, and I'll keep you informed as the review progresses,' came Emer's response.

After the meeting, when I was back in my room, I was noted by my 1:1 nurse to be anxious, sitting up suddenly in my bed and sighing.

'Everything OK?' she asked.

'I'm worried about the way the meeting went.'

'I'm sure you've nothing to be worried about.'

'Oh, come ON!' I exclaimed, exasperated at her attempt to fob me off.

'What do you mean by that?'

'Nothing,' I responded. 'I'm talking to myself.'

'I want to see my children, you know,' I added a few minutes later.

'Well, Tusla will be liaising with Emer next week and a visit will be arranged after that.'

After next week! I thought in despair, and I said nothing

further to my nurse. She noted then that I was '*lying in bed facing window* [. . .] *pleasant in interactions* [. . .] *guarded and at times monosyllabic in answers*'.

Later that day, I was invited into the TV room (which had been vacated by the other patients) to meet a psychologist from the psychosis service connected to the hospital. She was accompanied by Dr Omicron, the psychiatrist who had conducted two interviews with me the previous week. Our interaction lasted approximately fifteen minutes and was to be the only time in the more than twelve weeks I spent as an in-patient in 2015 that I chatted in person to any kind of psychologist or psychotherapist (as opposed to a psychiatrist). I remember her asking me a few questions about John, and expressing sympathy for my loss, before handing me a leaflet about cognitive behavioural therapy and some information about a CBT course that would be available to me once I was discharged from hospital. 'He must have been a great support to you,' I recall her saying. I was touched by her compassion and I felt a strong urge to tell her more about John and our relationship. It was on the tip of my tongue to respond that yes, John had been a great support to me, but that *I* had also been a great support to *him*. But by the time I had formulated my response, they had already departed, and I was left feeling deflated. What had seemed like an opportunity to form a meaningful human connection had vanished.

*

The Episode

My resemblance to Gregor Samsa when he awoke from anxious dreams was not limited to the *fact* of the transformation. When Gregor examined his body from his lying position in bed, he was repulsed by what he saw: a brown, arched abdomen; numerous, pitifully thin legs; an itchy part of his abdomen entirely covered in white spots. In my case, it was my bowels that repelled me, and the realization to my horror within a few days of entering the locked ward that I was constipated. This was no ordinary constipation: I had no recollection whatsoever of when I had last had a 'movement' – it was definitely weeks and might even have been back in September when I was first in hospital. Along with the shock of realization came a physical change that was impossible for me to ignore: a foul-smelling seepage into my pants that I attempted to stem with wads of toilet paper whenever I had the opportunity.

On Saturday, 24 October, I was on my way back from the courtyard with my 1:1 nurse when I rushed to the toilet.

'What just happened there?' the nurse wanted to know when I re-joined her.

'I needed to use the toilet,' I mumbled. The nurse seemed dissatisfied with my response, so I added: 'I'm constipated.'

'How long has that been going on for?' she enquired.

'Five days,' I said, panicking. I knew that it had been many multiples of five days, but I was too defeated and too ashamed to admit that, along with all my other failings and humiliations, I had no idea whatsoever of how long it had been.

Metamorphosis

The nurse arranged for me to be examined by the same female psychiatrist I had met in the mental health facility in late August when I was first prescribed antipsychotic medication. I told this doctor, too, that the constipation had been a problem for five or six days, careful to remain consistent with what I had said to my nurse.

'Do you have pain?' the doctor asked.

'No.'

'Bloating or discomfort?'

'No,' I answered again, all of which was true that day when the doctor asked me.

'You need to improve your diet and your fluid intake,' the doctor advised, and I was noted to be '*agreeable with that*'. I had already been taking a 'stool softener', sodium docusate, since after I was re-hospitalized – perhaps all long-stay patients were given this, I don't know – and now the doctor prescribed lactulose, 15ml, to be taken once daily as needed. But to my recollection, I was given lactulose only once, probably because I would never again admit to being constipated.

There was at least one further similarity between me and Gregor Samsa at this time: while Gregor was lying in his locked bedroom examining his body and trying to figure out what was wrong with him, he could hear people talking about him from the other room. Like me, he cared a lot about what others, and particularly his immediate family,

The Episode

thought about his predicament and he was highly agitated at what he heard. He could hear his mother calling him ('The soft voice!'), but when he attempted to answer, Gregor was startled by his own distorted and barely comprehensible voice. He also heard his work manager coming to visit, demanding to know why he was neglecting his commercial duties 'in a truly unheard of manner'. Gregor was 'beside himself' with agitation at the mean insinuations but, like me, he was dismayed to realize that he was unable to make himself understood by people who were standing a mere few metres away from him. 'Did you understand a single word?' the Manager asked Gregor's parents, while Gregor listened through his bedroom door. 'That was an animal's voice,' the Manager said.

For a long time, when my mother showed up for her daily visits, I felt shock at her ability to physically enter this other world that I was inhabiting, and disbelief that she could possibly still be loyal to me. I remember experiencing extreme agitation one evening at the thought of her hearing about my confession, and at the prospect of her giving up on me altogether. Eventually, all I felt when my mother appeared by my bedside was despair at my inability to explain my predicament to her. I derived no pleasure from her visits because I was unable to tell her about my constipation, or about the terrible mess I had got myself into with Dr Alpha and with Tusla.

I also talked to the children most evenings from the one

phone available to patients on the corridor of the ward, and every time I heard their voices, my heart broke into little pieces.

'When will you be home?' my older son asked me over and over again.

'Will you be back for Hallowe'en?' his little brother would ask in his squeaky voice.

'I don't know, sweetheart,' I responded every time, aware that the nursing staff were listening and possibly taking notes, and that the other patients on the ward could hear me too.

'Will you be home for my birthday?' my older son started to enquire in early November.

Later it became, 'Will you be home for Christmas?' and at every question I felt a stab of remorse at my inability to provide adequate answers and at the thought of my poor fatherless little children, their grief still fresh, with no mother to wave them goodbye at the school gates and nobody to hold them tight as they fell asleep at night.

On Wednesday, 28 October, social worker Emer came to meet me on the ward. As every professional always did when they interviewed me, she had a 'witness' with her – my 1:1 nurse for the day.

'How are you today?' Emer asked as I struggled to bring her face into focus.

'I'm fine,' I told her.

'Are you having contact with your family?'

The Episode

'Yes, my mother is visiting every day and I talk to the children every evening on the phone,' I answered.

'I'm here about the inter-agency family meeting with Tusla. It won't be scheduled for this week, unfortunately. It should take place at some point next week.'

'OK,' I said, feeling crushed by the knowledge that it would be at least next week before I would see the children.

'Your mother will be attending the meeting, and your brother from the US.'

I was surprised to hear that this brother would be travelling from so far away, and wondered silently whether a meeting about me and my children might also involve me.

Still the questioning continued. I was reviewed on 30 October on a ward round by a team consisting of Drs Alpha and Beta, social worker Emer and two members of the nursing staff, and once again by Dr Alpha in my room on both 1 and 2 November. No new incriminating details were elicited from me during these reviews, according to the records from this time, which also contain the first small hints that I was starting to improve.

'I'm feeling a little bit brighter,' I told Dr Alpha on one of her visits to my bedside.

'Any ideas, thoughts or plans of harming yourself, your children or anyone else?'

'None,' I responded wearily. 'I love my sons and I would never harm them.'

Metamorphosis

'Are you having much contact with them?'

'Yes, I phone them every night and I enjoy talking to them. The most important thing for me now is to meet them. It's been three weeks since I've seen them, and we've never been separated for this long.'

Dr Alpha nodded in response.

'I miss them terribly and I want to see them,' I persisted. 'When can I see my children?'

'Well, Tusla's inter-agency meeting is taking place the coming Friday and Emer will give you feedback after that,' Dr Alpha responded, shutting down the conversation.

As the days of early November rolled by, my constipation became more distressing to me, and the associated difficulties more repulsive and more shameful. It had become difficult to walk, and I developed a heavy, uncomfortable, wide-legged gait as I strolled the corridors of the locked ward and went for short walks with my 1:1 nurse in the hospital courtyard. The only person to comment on my condition was the close friend from my student days in Germany who visited from Berlin in early November and whose perceptiveness and unique candour are two of the things I love most about her. She and I went for a slow stroll in the hospital grounds, trailed by my nurse. I remember my friend sharing what she had seen earlier in the day at my house when she had visited my mother and children, and I recall being barely able to respond to her in my zombie-like state.

The Episode

'Bernie is overly protective of the boys and won't let them outside to play,' she told me, painting a scene that I could envisage only too well: my mother's disciplinarian streak always came to the fore in the presence of young children, perhaps because she had been a primary school teacher all her working life.

'Do you understand that you're not helping yourself by not taking your medication and by leaving the hospital grounds?' my friend asked.

'Yes, I understand,' I replied, stunned that my friend, who had arrived in Ireland the previous day, seemed to have been briefed about my medication compliance.

'Warum läufst du so komisch?' she asked suddenly. I shrugged my shoulders in response, before agreeing wordlessly with her speculation that it was probably the effects of the medication that were causing me to walk so strangely.

Long after the events of 2015, after I had read my records and learned that psychotic depression was the diagnosis I had been given in hospital, I came across an academic article entitled 'Distinguishing Psychotic Depression from Melancholia'. I was stunned by what I read in that article: all my symptoms were staring back at me from the pages: delusions, 'morbid' cognitions ('involving guilt and a sense of deserving punishment'), and even constipation. Further symptoms identified in the article as presenting with greater severity in psychotic depression while also being present in other types of melancholia were recognizable to me both from memory and from the clinical language used in my patient record: psychomotor disturbance/retardation, appetite and weight loss, terminal insomnia, and loss of interest/anhedonia (the inability to feel pleasure in normally pleasurable activities).

No explanation is offered in the article for the high incidence of constipation in psychotic depression apart from a statement that it is 'not a consequence of medication'. However, I can put forward a theory of my own based on my personal experience and on what I've since read about the impact of trauma on mind and body. I see constipation as a symptom, along with insomnia and loss of appetite, of what is sometimes called the 'reptilian' brain shutting down in situations of severe stress. 'It is amazing,' Bessel van der Kolk writes in *The Body Keeps the Score*, 'how many psychological problems involve difficulties with sleep, appetite, touch, digestion, and arousal.' In his discussion of the brain's response to trauma, van der Kolk draws on the three-part description of the brain drawn up by neuroscientist Paul MacLean. When we go into fight-or-flight mode against 'real' or 'imaginary' assailants, our emotional brain (or what van der Kolk refers to as the 'smoke detector') goes into overdrive, triggering strong visceral sensations and flooding the system with stress hormones. Meanwhile, the other two parts of the brain – the reptilian brain, which manages the basic 'housekeeping' functions of the body, and the frontal cortex, the rational, monitoring, 'watchtower' part – switch off and retreat

The Episode

offline. This reads like a description of what happened during the breakdown of my mind and body in 2015, and of why it was no coincidence that my 'reptilian' brain kicked back into gear with the leakage from my bowel at exactly the same time as the rational, thinking part woke up and began to survey the carnage caused over the previous months by my overactive 'smoke detector'.

16

This Hospital Does Not Dispense Sweets

The road to recovery was neither linear nor continuous; it was fitful, painful and slow. The experience was also intensely lonely. To anyone observing me stretched out on my hospital bed, I might have looked the same as I always had since re-entering hospital on 9 October, but inside the bony cavity of my skull the landscape was changing. My delusional guilt over my imagined crime was diminishing in intensity, and with it the depression from which I had been suffering since late August. Yet it yielded not to happiness, but to despair over the foolishness of my utterances and over the misunderstandings and hopelessness that characterized my situation in the hospital.

The records of my conversations with nursing staff and their observations of me in late October and early November hint at the transformation I was undergoing. When asked how I was doing, I generally responded that I was 'OK' or that I was starting to feel 'better'. There were only a couple of occasions when I revealed a little of what I was actually

The Episode

feeling about my circumstances. One of these was to 'Johanna', the pretty middle-aged nurse with the kind face, beautiful skin and soft cashmere sweaters who was starting to win my trust, not least because she was someone I saw on a semi-regular basis, unlike most of her nursing colleagues. '*Spent long periods this evening laying in bed staring at the ceiling,*' Johanna wrote of me on 4 November. '*Rested in bed, began to talk.*'

'I feel so depressed I don't want to live any more!' I said, referring to the seemingly open-ended nature of my confinement and to the ongoing separation from my children.

'What about the boys?' Johanna asked.

'Well, I don't see them anyway, do I?' I retorted angrily.

'Do you have a suicide plan here in the hospital?'

'No, I don't have a suicide plan!' I snapped back at her.

While Johanna noted following this conversation that I remained '*flat in affect*' and '*also angry in affect*', I interpret this flash of irritation as a small sign that I was starting to kick back at the bleakness of my situation and speak up about my needs, although my efforts in this respect remained feeble at best. There was another occasion too from this time when one of the constantly changing cast of 1:1 nurses shadowing my every move noted that I had '*spent some time on the bed interacting well in conversation*'.

'Am I ever going to be let out of here?' I asked the nurse after I had spoken to her for a few moments in a 'normal' fashion about John and the two children.

'Of course you are,' she responded.

'I don't like having a special nurse with me all the time, you know,' I added a few minutes later.

'It's for your safety,' the nurse responded, and I could think of nothing to say in reply.

'I find it difficult to sleep here,' I said finally. 'It's because of the lack of physical activity.' Since being placed on 'special' observation, I had been led like a prison inmate once a day into a tiny internal courtyard adorned with fitness equipment where I would walk my miserable rounds for twenty minutes before being chaperoned back to the ward. I hated that courtyard with its pathetic shrubs and sad pieces of gym equipment, not least because it was a wholly inadequate exercise space for someone who had thrived on hiking and jogging and vigorous physical workouts when well. 'That courtyard is way too small for me to walk around,' I complained to the nurse. 'And the gym equipment is crap! You know most of the gym equipment in the outdoors is a joke?'

I was also starting at this time to take a small interest in things around me that had previously given me pleasure. I was beginning to enjoy food again and I caught myself looking forward to mealtimes, especially because meals on the locked ward were tasty and nutritious, far superior to what was served up on other wards, a peculiarity that I heard other patients commenting on. Occasionally, too, I was observed to be reading. My mother had brought me a book – *Pride and Prejudice*, an old favourite of hers – but it was almost

The Episode

impossible for me to forget my worries for long enough to focus on the words in front of me, and I found television to be a better distraction. I hadn't made it home in time for Hallowe'en as my children had hoped, and on the evening of 31 October, while my friends took them trick-or-treating on the streets of our neighbourhood, I was noted to have *'watched most of the rugby match in* [the] *corridor, interacting little with staff or clients during* [the] *game'*. This was the final of the 2015 Rugby World Cup, and I remember being enthralled by New Zealand's spectacular performance, while reflecting sadly on how elated John would have been to see his beloved Wales reach the quarter-finals and, better still, beat its old foe, England, in the group stage, contributing to England's elimination. (I would find myself musing in a similar vein a few months later when the football club he supported, Leicester City, won the English Premier League for the first time in the club's history, and the Welsh national football team reached the semi-finals of the European championship, having failed to even qualify for a major tournament in fifty-eight years – almost exactly the entire duration of John's life.) I had always enjoyed watching sport of almost any kind, and now that the TV was no longer a source of terror for me, I found myself drawn to it. A few days later I was observed to be *'quite animated'* watching a football match and *'at one point let out a big sigh when a goal was missed'*. I was quoted as saying that I didn't follow football, *'however whenever it was on she would "get really into the game"'*. Getting 'really into' a sports event was a sure sign that I was recovering, not only from my episode of mental collapse but also from the crippling grief that had sullied my enjoyment of almost everything following John's death in April.

I don't know what exactly caused the seismic shift in my internal topography as I was languishing on the locked ward and pining for my children in early November. Perhaps it was simply the passage of time and the opportunity to take a rest from the demands of my life outside the hospital. An alternative, or perhaps additional, explanation could be that there may be a limit to the number and range of subjects that a human mind can fret over simultaneously. I have often wondered since then whether my capacity to ruminate was so exhausted by the concrete fears assailing me about what the future held for me and my family that there was simply no room left for obsessions about an imagined crime in the past. As my brain shifted focus from 'insane' to 'real-world' preoccupations, and the so-called 'positive' symptoms of my psychosis loosened their hold over me, the 'negative' symptoms – loss of appetite, insomnia, inability to focus, anhedonia – also lost their intensity and gradually disappeared.

Medication almost certainly played a role in my nascent recovery. Following my re-admission, and particularly after I was transferred to the locked ward, Dr Alpha and her team appear to have thrown the proverbial kitchen sink at me in

The Episode

their prescribing of psychiatric drugs. Olanzapine, the antipsychotic drug that I had taken for over six weeks from late August, had been reintroduced at a dose of 10mg every night, and my venlafaxine dose increased from 225mg to 300mg every morning. This brought to a total of six the number of psychotropic drugs I was taking – two antipsychotics, two antidepressants, one sleeping tablet and one benzodiazepine. Even at the time, I was aware that this was a dizzying array of medication. The sheer number of pills that I was required to swallow twice daily frightened me, especially as someone who had never been convinced that tablets held the solution to psychological distress. I knew the names and types of drugs I was ingesting because, along the way, I had been handed information leaflets about most if not all of them. I was aware too of the dosages because 'meds' were always dispensed by two nurses – one to read aloud the medication card once a patient had shuffled to the top of the queue snaking up the corridor to the nurses' station, and one to measure out the pills into small, conical paper cups to be handed to the waiting patients. I had little idea, though, of whether the doses were big or small, or how the different drugs interacted with one another and what the risks associated with taking such a seemingly vast quantity of medication might be.

As it turns out, the doses *were* very high, and in addition to the deadening cognitive and emotional effects, the risks to my physical health were considerable. According to two

This Hospital Does Not Dispense Sweets

documents in my patient record, my daily dosage of antipsychotic medication exceeded the recommended maximum by 12.5 per cent and was therefore '*unlicensed*' and '*off-label*'. In combination with the two antidepressants I was taking, this meant there was '*a risk of development of long QT* [irregular heart rhythm], *lowered threshold for seizures and possibility of development of increased blood pressure*', all of which required '*careful monitoring of blood pressure, sodium levels, and regular ECG*'. I remember the daily temperature and blood-pressure monitoring, the occasional blood tests and the repeated electrocardiograms (ECGs). To begin with, I thought that the ECGs were intended to fool me because the machine kept breaking down and the sensors attached to my skin to detect the electrical signals produced by my heart kept peeling off. I also recall feeling apprehensive that once I lifted my top to have the sensors attached, the nurse conducting the test might notice a bulge in my stomach and ask about 'movements'. But this never happened, and eventually, I realized that the tests were real, although the equipment *was* faulty, and I was never informed why they were being conducted in the first place.

If I was asked to identify one drug that possibly made a difference for me it would have to be risperidone, because as early as one week after I started taking it, my delusional guilt started to wane. In his book *Psychiatric Drugs Explained*, psychiatrist and academic David Healy writes that when antipsychotics work, 'to observers, it often appears that the

The Episode

voices or delusions seem to lose their grip, and the person seems less likely to act on them after some days or weeks on the drugs. [. . .] More often than not, however, questioning reveals that the hallucinations or delusions have not entirely disappeared. It is more usual that takers of antipsychotics will still have their voices or some of their ideas, but they are less worried by them.' This is exactly what happened to me remarkably soon after I started taking risperidone: my delusional belief didn't disappear overnight, it just became less powerful, and I was no longer particularly bothered about whether my sons had ingested my pills or not.

On more than one occasion, I queried the amount of medication I was taking with the medical team treating me. The rationale for so many drugs was explained to me a number of times – the team had been noticing a change in my mood, I was told. I had more luck when I questioned the need to continue taking a benzodiazepine and a sleeping tablet every night, and Dr Alpha agreed to cut back the clonazepam tablet and to stop the regular zopiclone. '*Patient describes oversedation*,' she wrote into my medication chart.

Every time I asked when I would see my children, I was told that the decision rested with Tusla. I learned that the interagency meeting would take place in my home on the morning of Friday, 6 November while the children were at school, and that it would be attended by Orlaith from Tusla, Dr Beta and social worker Emer, and by my mother and my brother

This Hospital Does Not Dispense Sweets

who lived in the US. I, however, would not be present. When my brother came to visit on the evening of 5 November, I asked whether he thought it strange that a meeting of this kind would not involve me. 'No, it's not strange at all,' he responded, and I felt acutely the pain of having apparently forfeited the right to participate in decisions around my children's care.

On the morning of 6 November, while waiting to learn the outcome of the gathering in my house, I was led into a multidisciplinary team meeting to find Dr Gamma chairing it. She was the psychiatrist whom I had last seen in my house with nurse Sue exactly four weeks previously, and seeing her now reminded me of the distressing circumstances of my re-admission.

'How would you rate your mood between one and ten?' Dr Gamma asked me at the start of the meeting.

'It's five, or maybe six,' I said, hoping to make myself agreeable to her and to the rest of the team, which included social worker Emer, three nurses, and Dr Beta, who was typing up a record of the meeting into a laptop propped up on his knees.

'That's an improvement, isn't it?' Dr Gamma commented, and I agreed that it was. *'Feels that things have improved for her during the last week,'* the notes of the meeting state. *'Objectively it appears to be the case [. . .] eating and sleeping well.'*

'And how was your mental state when you left the

The Episode

hospital and went to the quarry and your sons' school?' Dr Gamma asked.

I gazed uncomfortably at the panel of six. I knew there was something wrong with the question, and I spent some moments trying to figure out what it was and whether it would be wise to correct it. But I lacked the lucidity and the self-confidence to point out that I had not, in fact, visited my children's school the day I left the hospital three weeks previously. 'It's difficult for me to talk about this,' I mumbled instead.

'What about the thoughts you had at that time, of harming yourself and your children and acting on those thoughts?'

Trying to be as honest as I could – after all I *had* looked at cars and trains and the quarry face and contemplated suicide in a vague and abstract way – I gathered up all my strength to state clearly (and the record quotes me verbatim): 'I had no real intent to act on those thoughts. Anyway, they were only ever in relation to myself, never to the boys. I never had a plan.'

'Why did you never express these thoughts when the team visited you at home or at other meetings?' Dr Gamma asked. Once again, I felt tripped up by Dr Gamma's question. The 'thoughts' she had just mentioned were not at all the same thoughts that had plagued me while I was still at home, which had related to the imagined crime of medicating my children. The correct answer to Dr Gamma's question would have been to say: 'The reason I never expressed the "thoughts" you are referring to is because I never had thoughts of wanting to harm myself or my children when I was at home, and I never had them in the hospital either.' But the issue was so complex and the confusion so complete that it was far beyond my limited cognitive capacities to set the record straight. As I considered how best to answer Dr Gamma's question, and as I gazed at Dr Beta's fingertips hovering over the keyboard awaiting my response, I was also acutely aware that anything I said might influence the outcome of Tusla's inter-agency meeting later that morning, on which any reunion with my children depended.

'It's not an easy subject to talk about,' I said finally.

After a further pause, Dr Gamma changed the subject: 'Have you any worries now?'

'I'm very worried that I will never be able to see my boys again,' I blurted out. 'I'm worried that the boys will be taken from me!'

'Well, the aim of our treatment plan is to have you discharged as soon as you're well enough and for you to return home to live with your boys. And once you're well enough, a supervised family meeting can also be arranged,' Dr Gamma explained, and it was noted that I was '*happy*' with this response.

'What about your thoughts in relation to having given your medication to the boys and the change in their academic performance? Are those thoughts still present now?' Dr Gamma asked.

The Episode

I hesitated again before answering as carefully and accurately as possible, 'They're not as intense. Anyway, I'll blank them out when I meet the boys.'

Later that afternoon, Emer visited me on the ward to brief me about the Tusla meeting.

'A contingency plan will be drawn up around childcare arrangements, providing respite for your mother,' she said.

'Will they be allowed to visit me now?' I asked.

'It's hoped that a visit can be organized for next week. I'll accompany you and the boys for the visit, which will take place in the family room on the ground floor. I'll discuss it further with you on Monday.'

'Thank you,' I said, hiding my disappointment that I would not be seeing the boys at the weekend as I had hoped.

When my brother visited me over the weekend, I told him I was being prevented from seeing my children.

'The doctors and social workers seem to think I'm some kind of danger to the boys,' I said.

'Well, if you talk to them about suicidal and homicidal thoughts,' my brother responded, 'they *will* see you as a risk, you know.' I wondered who had told him about my disclosures, and who else had been briefed about them.

'So you know about the day I left the hospital?' I asked carefully.

'Of course we know about it!' he exclaimed. 'We were

worried sick about you.' When I said nothing in response, he added: 'You *do* have a family who loves you, you know?' and I gave a weak nod to indicate that I knew.

What he said next about the nature of my breakdown was far more helpful; in fact, it was the single most helpful thing that anyone said to me during my entire period in hospital.

'It's an episode,' he pronounced more than once during the several visits he paid me over the weekend of 7/8 November. 'An episode has a beginning, a middle and an end,' he said over and over, almost like a mantra. 'You're now in the middle – and the middle is horrendous – but episodes always end, and this *will* end.'

No mental health professional ever said anything remotely similar in all the months I spent being treated by them. It would have helped if they had. As it was, my brother's mantra gave me hope. And it turned out to be true.

On the evening of Monday, 9 November, a friend showed up out of the blue. I know the exact date because the conversation I had immediately after her visit is captured in my patient record. It was at a time when I was allowed '*staff accompanied access to coffee shop, hospital grounds/open garden*', so my friend and I went downstairs to the cafeteria together, shadowed by Johanna, the attractive, middle-aged nurse who had been attempting over the previous weeks to establish a rapport with me. For the first time since early August, I shed a few tears as my friend talked about her father's

The Episode

sudden death when she and her brother were teenagers, and about how her mother had brought them up on her own, as well as running the family farm single-handedly. As my friend spoke, and as I compared myself to her mother, I thought about my own inadequacies and wept tears of self-reproach and failure.

One of the strangest aspects of my experience since early August had been my inability to cry, and a tiny piece of me thawed with those tears. After my friend had gone, and nurse Johanna and I had returned to the ward, I fell into conversation with her. I cried some more as I told her about my feelings of guilt – not pathological guilt for a crime I had never committed, just 'normal', if misplaced, guilt for my breakdown and for not having had the strength to hold myself together for my children's sake. 'I just fell apart,' I said to her, according to her notes. As I opened up a little more, I shared some of my lingering suspicions with her. Paranoia had pre-dated my delusional thoughts back in August, and it was also the last symptom to disappear entirely. Ever since I had been transferred to my new bed on the locked ward, I had been noticing doctors and nurses entering and leaving the room next to mine. I had only ever seen one occupant of that room, but the medical personnel would go in there even when that patient was in the smoking room or sitting beside me on the ward, watching TV. Nurses would carry in meals and return with bedpans and empty trays, and entire teams would suddenly arrive and crowd into the room unannounced.

This Hospital Does Not Dispense Sweets

I was convinced that this was an elaborate charade to deceive me into believing that there were two patients in the room next to mine, and I confided in Johanna that I knew all about the pretence going on next door:

'There's only one patient in there,' I told her, 'and for some reason they're pretending there's two.'

Once I started to open up, I felt unable to stop until I had told her about everything that was puzzling me on the ward, including the fact that I had walked in on my room-mate a number of times chatting in an empty room and hurrying to hide something. 'Another thing I've noticed is that all the other patients on this ward have mobile phones,' I told Johanna. 'I'm the only one who doesn't, and you just don't see it.'

Finally, I shared my belief that some of the pills I was being given at night-time were sweets: 'They're pink,' I said, 'they have a sweet taste and they melt as soon as I put them in my mouth.'

At that week's team meeting a few days later, after we had dispensed with the usual questions about 'thoughts of harm' and how I was feeling on a scale from one to ten, Dr Alpha brought up my conversation with Johanna. She repeated my words back at me as I squirmed uncomfortably on my seat. Her comments are not recorded in my patient record, but I remember them very well:

'There are *two* patients in the room next to yours,' Dr Alpha stated, while I hung my head in shame and listened to the idiocy of my words.

The Episode

'No patient on this ward has access to their own phone,' she continued.

'And,' she concluded with a mirthless smile, 'this hospital does not dispense sweets to patients.'

As I heard the ramblings of my still-distressed mind repeated back to me, the last traces of the insanity that had produced them disappeared in a puff of humiliation. I felt a surge of hatred towards Dr Alpha and her entire team, including Johanna, by whom I felt betrayed, and I pictured the derision that would rain down on me if they were ever to find out that I had been constipated for longer than I could remember.

17

Supervised Visits

I met my children for the first time in over a month at 3 p.m. on Wednesday, 11 November. It is difficult to describe what being reunited with them under these circumstances felt like. The longest, and indeed only, time we had ever been separated up to this point was four nights a year and a half previously, when I had attended a training course in Berlin, reliving some of the happy freedoms of my student years, while John had kept house in reciprocation for the sports- and music-filled weekends he would occasionally spend with his friends in the UK as the children grew bigger and easier for one of us to manage alone. What I remember most about the reunion was the sensation of seeing my sons 'objectively' for the first time, almost as a benign stranger would, and of being overwhelmed by how adorable they were. They struck me as extraordinarily beautiful, and I gazed in wonder at their glowing skin and wide smiles until my brain adjusted to the intensity of being back in the company of my two gorgeous, funny, boisterous boys again.

Even at the time, I was aware that the separation probably

The Episode

hadn't been enforced for therapeutic reasons, and that we had been prevented from meeting due to other, 'risk'-related, concerns. But not seeing my children for four weeks, heartbreaking as it had been for all of us, seems to have had a therapeutic effect on me, especially as the root cause of my distress had been my belief that my sons were irreparably damaged. The four weeks had given me time to divert my thoughts elsewhere, to topics which could hardly be described as 'happy', but which were nonetheless less distressing to me. When I met the children now, I could see that apart from the fact that their hair was too long and that someone had dressed them in ugly sweatpants that I would never have bought for them, there was nothing at all wrong with them and there was therefore nothing for me to feel guilty about.

Social worker Emer had told me in advance of the visit that she and my mother would both be present for the duration, and that she herself would be there in a 'non-judgemental' capacity. I stared at her when she said this, instinctively feeling that her use of the word 'non-judgemental' was disingenuous. I also remember wondering aloud to Emer how the children and I would spend the visit. They were not at an age where we could just sit around chatting for an hour, so I suggested bringing along a jigsaw from the ward, and Emer agreed that this was a good idea. Her record of the supervised visit starts with the sentence: '*M greeted her children in the foyer* [. . .] *and was spontaneously smiling during this interaction.*' Then all five of us – me, my mother, my two children and Emer – went together to the family room, where I and the children sat over the jigsaw puzzle and kicked a ball around in an adjacent courtyard.

'When will you be coming home?' my younger son asked me during a break from the play.

'Whenever they let me,' I responded, trying to keep the mood light.

'Will you be home for my birthday?' his older brother asked.

'Whenever Mammy comes home, we'll celebrate your birthday then,' my mother interjected, and I gave her a weak smile of gratitude for providing an answer that seemed to placate the boy.

Emer noted that I *'brightened when engaging with the children in their play'* and that, after we had gone to the canteen together, I *'purchased some snacks and sat with the boys for a period'* and *'was observed to be chatting with them'*. She also noted that my mother provided me with an update *'around the practicalities of caring for the boys, e.g., who would be bringing them to a number of upcoming friends' birthday parties'*. The visit concluded when my mother's friend called to bring them all home, and I returned to the ward with Johanna. *'On return from the family visit,'* my patient record states, *'M appeared bright initially, smiling appropriately with other clients on the unit and walking with an upright posture.'* Later that evening, I *'declined to go on the evening walk with other clients on the unit'*, reporting that I *'wanted to be alone'*.

*

The Episode

Emer had informed me that she would be available for another visit from my sons the following Wednesday or Thursday, and I agreed to discuss the logistics with my mother. However, I was aggrieved, and even offended, by Emer's insistence that the visits needed to be not only scheduled, but also supervised, by her. I had already told the team truthfully and multiple times that I never planned to harm my children in any way, and I couldn't imagine what they thought might happen if I met my sons alone – or rather, alone with my ninety-year-old mother, who would always be accompanying them on their visits. I was also starting to wonder what authority Emer or anyone else had to prevent us from meeting whenever we chose to.

'Is there some kind of barring order against me?' I asked her, two days after the first visit.

'No, there isn't. Why do you ask?'

'Well, why do you have to be there during the visits?'

'I'm there as a support to you because you're on this ward, which is a safe environment. And it's because of the distressing thoughts you had about ending your own and your boys' lives.'

I gazed at Emer, unsure of how to respond. 'I'm not currently having those thoughts,' was all I could think of to say.

When Emer wrote her entry that day, she noted that the question of why she was joining the visits with my children *'had been discussed with M by myself this morning and on two previous occasions prior to her visit with the children this week'*. Emer was right – it *had* been discussed with me 'this morning' at a multidisciplinary team meeting attended by a record *eight* professionals: Drs Alpha and Beta, social worker Emer, nurse Sue, whose presence always evoked a nervous response in me, an occupational therapist, a nurse from the ward, along with a student nurse and a student social worker (both unknown to me). I remember the conversation at the meeting very well, and the notes entered on to the MHIS corroborate my recollection of what was said:

'How would you rate your mood on a scale of one to ten?' Dr Alpha asked.

'Five out of ten.'

'Have you any thoughts of harming yourself or anyone else?'

'No. I've none.'

'Do you have any questions that you would like to ask us?'

'Yes, I do have a question. Why does a social worker have to be present when I'm meeting my children?'

The record of the meeting states that Emer '*explained the rationale behind this*'. I don't remember exactly what that 'rationale' was, but it had something to do with 'my thoughts' and the fact that I was on the locked ward – even though I had seen other patients on this ward receiving unsupervised visits from their children. The record states that I appeared '*to be defensive and puzzled about this position and somewhat angry*'. The rest of the exchange went as follows:

The Episode

'It won't be for ever,' Emer said.

'Really?' I interjected.

'I hope it doesn't make a difference my being there in the room with you,' the social worker added, giving me an innocuous smile as I felt my temper rising.

'Yes, actually, it very much *does* make a difference having somebody in the room observing me when my children are visiting,' I retorted, surprising myself with the forcefulness of my response.

When I returned to my bed following that team meeting, I was shocked at my own display of anger, but now I see it as an indication that, as my recovery progressed, I was starting to fight back ever so slightly. Alas, I never felt brave enough to broach the subject of constipation. The seepage into my pants was worsening, and I found myself rushing to the bathroom ten, fifteen, even twenty times a day, to try to stem it with wads of bunched-up toilet paper. I didn't have enough underwear (or enough of any kind of clothes), having left home so precipitously on 9 October, so I had to wash out the few items in my possession as often as possible and hang them over the radiator in my room, hoping that they would be dry by morning and that no one would ask what I was doing. As for owning up to having been constipated for so long, this seemed like just as big a hurdle to overcome and just as impossible to resolve as all the other misunderstandings I was facing. The only difference now was that rather

Supervised Visits

than needing to *unsay* something that I had said during my breakdown, I needed to *say* something that had been left *unsaid* all this time. As I searched in shame and desperation for a solution, I was at a loss as to whom to confide in. While I have little doubt now that the matter would have been dealt with sensitively, at the time I pictured myself being chastised by Dr Alpha for having 'lied' about the matter, and it seemed safest to say nothing at all.

As mid-November approached, entries into my patient record show that my cognitive state was continuing to improve.

'Do you still think everybody else on the ward has a mobile phone?' nurse Johanna asked me on 11 November.

'Yes,' I responded, but after a short pause, I added, 'No, maybe not.'

I remember sitting in the communal area at this time, occasionally watching TV on my own or in the company of – but not conversing with – other patients. I recall being transfixed by the news in the days following the Paris attacks of 13 November, when Islamist terrorists attacked the Bataclan concert hall and the Stade de France during an international football game, and being eventually asked by one of the nurses to turn off the television because the news was upsetting the other patients. I also remember that same male nurse trying to draw me out, almost pleading with me to tell him what was troubling me. It felt like he was attempting to ascertain what was *actually* wrong with me, and it

The Episode

was on the tip of my tongue to mention constipation. But I couldn't find the words to begin.

'I'm fine. I'm improving,' I told him.

A second supervised family visit took place on Wednesday, 18 November. I was escorted to the family room by a member of the nursing staff, and I was met there by Emer, the children and my mother. When I arrived in the room, my sons were playing with beanbags and a bicycle. I chatted to them and then to my mother, who went through the schedule for the boys over the coming days – who would be collecting them from school, whose houses they would be visiting and so on. In her notes of the visit, Emer wrote that I '*spent a short period with the children in the courtyard area and then sat with them to have a drink and cake*'. As we walked together to the canteen, she noted, my older son '*held hands with M*', while his brother walked behind with Emer herself, '*playing "jumping on the squares in the carpet!"*'. When it came time for them to depart, I was '*observed to hug* [the children] *goodbye*'.

It must have been directly after this visit when Emer remarked to me that it was not appropriate for my mother and me to be discussing childcare arrangements in front of the children.

'It's not nice for them to hear those conversations,' she commented. 'Perhaps I should ask your mother to stop.'

I was unable to imagine what was wrong with our choice

of topic. 'Please don't ask her,' I said, while pondering the extraordinary juncture I had reached in my life when I was being told what I could and could not discuss in front of my children. 'I have to talk about these things when I meet my mother,' I added.

'Are you satisfied now that there's not a barring order against you?' Emer asked, changing the subject.

'I suppose so. But I still don't get why you need to accompany me on these visits.'

'This is as a support to you,' Emer said. 'And it's also based on the distressing thoughts you had prior to your re-admission.'

I said nothing at all to this, so Emer continued: 'You've been doing a good job organizing for the boys to be entertained during the visits, like asking for the football and checking that the books are suitable for their age. Well done!'

'Thank you,' I responded, attempting a smile.

'You do know that the visits won't continue to be accompanied indefinitely, don't you?'

'Yes,' I said, although I had been told nothing at all about how long the supervision arrangements were likely to remain in place.

'And that you will continue to recover.'

'Yes, I suppose so.'

18

Safety Planning

During the first half of November, my observation levels were gradually relaxed until, on 19 November, I was transferred back to the unlocked ward where I had been accommodated before going AWOL just over a month previously. Four days after the transfer, Emer introduced me to 'Cathy', the new Tusla social worker assigned to my case after Orlaith had concluded her work, following the inter-agency meeting attended by my US brother on 6 November. Cathy was younger than her predecessor and more prone to crack a smile. I also remember being struck by her peculiar use of the word 'piece' – used in place of 'aspect' or 'dimension' or 'element'. I had never heard it used this way before, although I have heard it lots of times in the years since and I am careful to avoid this usage myself. Over the following days and weeks, Cathy would refer to the 'parenting piece', or the 'safety piece', or the 'fostering piece', and my still fatigued brain would ponder the word 'piece' for a couple of seconds before grasping what she meant. Like some other care workers, she

Safety Planning

also had a habit of referring to me in my presence as 'Mum', which felt reductionist, patronizing and wrong.

'We have received some very serious reports about you,' I remember Cathy saying when she first met me on 23 November (although this part of the exchange is not captured in any medical or social work record now in my possession, unlike the rest of the conversation). 'Do you understand the gravity of those reports?'

'Yes,' I responded, feeling the colour rise to my face as I recalled the disastrous confessions I had made following my transfer to the locked ward.

'I'm part of the child welfare team,' Cathy informed me. 'My role is to carry out a continued assessment of the family's needs and to explore any potential supports required in the event of a phased discharge.'

'What kind of supports?' I asked.

'Well, engaging with a treatment plan could be one example. Or your sons might attend Barnardo's Children's Charity for bereavement work.'

I nodded that I understood.

'I will also be carrying out an assessment of risk to the children,' Cathy continued.

'Risk to the children?' I asked, my stomach tightening in fear. 'Why would you need to do that?'

'We know about the distressing thoughts you had before your admission, when you were unwell,' Cathy responded.

The Episode

'What thoughts?' I began, but the sceptical look on the social worker's face made me stop.

'I'll be meeting your children later this week and will inform you of the time and date,' she continued.

'I'm meeting them myself this Wednesday,' I said. I had been informed that the forthcoming visit would be unsupervised – probably because I was now on an unlocked ward – but that it would take place on the ward, rather than downstairs in the family room or the hospital canteen.

At the end of the meeting, Cathy instructed me: 'It is important that you don't discharge yourself without your doctors' advice.' I nodded to indicate that I understood.

It turns out that planning for what would happen if I went AWOL was top of Cathy's priority list when she took over my case. Emer noted that on the day she first met me, Cathy *'requested an inter-agency safety planning meeting to be held this week involving her team leader, the Gardaí and* [the] *treating team'*. The purpose of the meeting, Emer wrote in an internal email, was *'to formulate a proposed safety plan around the event that M is absent without leave from hospital'*. It was scheduled for Friday, 27 November, and I learned about it the previous day when Cathy called in to me on the ward to inform me that I would also be attending.

'The gardaí will be at your meeting with Tusla tomorrow,' a male nurse mentioned to me in passing later that day.

Safety Planning

'The guards?' I responded in consternation. 'Why the *guards?*'

'Well, that's what Tusla have told us,' he replied.

Following my introduction to Cathy, I was tormented by a new set of worries. I wondered what she had meant by 'assessment of risk to the children' and I fretted over the 'serious' reports about me received by Tusla. I wondered who would have written them – Dr Alpha? Emer? – and how many of the multiple self-incriminating things I had said during the acute stage of my breakdown might have been communicated to the agency. All the while, the nurses were pressing me to open up. *'Remains guarded on the ward. Not willing to engage much with staff* [. . .] *minimal interaction with staff* [. . .] *unwilling to engage with nursing staff at present,'* entry upon entry in my patient record from this time states. A stiffly worded entry from 25 November notes that *'it was outlined to M that her treatment would benefit from more of her input to staff on how she feels and what she's thinking'*. But I couldn't begin to explain to the nursing staff what was troubling me and so I limited myself to reporting that my mood was 'up and down' after seeing my sons – 'happy' that I had seen them but 'sad' that I was not at home with them.

On the morning of 27 November – the day of the 'safety planning' meeting – I was summoned to a team meeting chaired by Dr Gamma.

The Episode

'Do you have any worries?' she asked me as five other staff members looked on and Dr Beta typed up my responses.

'Well, my main worries are about the children and my discharge date. I'm actually almost back to myself but I'm unsure how to show you this.'

I waited to be told how I could show this, but my words were met with silence. 'I'm afraid I'll never get home!' I added, a pleading tone entering my voice.

'What about your thoughts around medication and your children?'

I looked around carefully at the six staff inspecting me. 'To be honest, I'm not sure if that ever happened,' I began slowly, and then, feeling a wave of relief at the truth of my words wash over me, I added with more conviction: 'I'm not worried about their academic performance or cognitive abilities any more really, although I only ever see them for a short time, so I suppose it's a bit hard to assess.'

'And your thoughts "if I should go they should go"? Do you still have those thoughts?'

I flinched inwardly at the question. It had been a number of weeks since I had last been asked directly about my 'homicidal and suicidal thoughts' and I had begun to hope that they'd been dismissed as the incoherent ramblings that they actually were. Now, forcing my over-medicated brain to choose my words carefully, I answered: 'I regret them,' by which I meant I regretted *saying* that I'd ever had such thoughts, although the record states that I '*regretted having*' the thoughts

Safety Planning

themselves. It also states that I was '*ashamed about the thoughts [I] had that day*' and that I '*found it difficult to talk about this area*'.

'We still think you're very sick,' Dr Gamma said suddenly, her face fixed in an expression of genuine compassion. 'How would you feel about starting a new medication?' I groaned silently at the thought of yet another drug at this late stage.

'Have you heard of lithium?' Dr Gamma asked.

'Yes,' I responded, aghast that she was proposing a drug which, as far as I knew, is taken long-term for chronic mental health conditions. 'I don't think I want to start it.'

'Well, why don't you have a read of this leaflet and have a think about it over the next few days?' she suggested. The record of the team meeting concludes by stating that I '*seemed open to this idea*'.

Later that day, I walked into Tusla's 'safety planning' meeting transfixed by dread. I scanned the faces of the professionals, looking for the police officer whose presence had been advertised to me. But all I could see were Dr Gamma, nurse Sue, social worker Emer, Tusla social worker Cathy, and her manager 'Bronagh', who glowered at me with what seemed like unconcealed dislike.

Before the meeting, I had requested a private discussion with Cathy. Her manager came too, and I asked what would happen to the children if my mother became ill while I was still in hospital. I was told that they would look at a respite

The Episode

foster placement. The safety planning meeting was briefed of this at the start, and that Cathy would meet me the following Monday to discuss this further. We were also informed that 'unfortunately' the liaison garda would not be attending the meeting, but that An Garda Síochána would be notified of the outcome. Then I was asked to leave the room and to wait outside.

Approximately thirty minutes later, I was brought back in. The conversation was led by Cathy, and it went as follows:

'If you ever leave this hospital again without permission, the gardaí will be notified and asked to assist in returning you. Do you understand?'

'Yes, I understand.'

'Do you have any questions?'

I mustered up my courage to ask, 'When will I be allowed to return home to my children?'

'Tusla's recommendation is that you will not have unsupervised care of your children at this point and the gardaí will be informed of this.'

'Will I ever return to parenting my children without Tusla being involved?' I asked, becoming aware of a tremor in my voice.

'As your illness resolves, it's Tusla's goal that the children will return to your care. But we have safety concerns around the serious nature of your thoughts. Do you understand?'

I nodded that I understood.

Safety Planning

'Any further questions?'

'No, I've no further questions,' I said quietly.

On returning to the ward, I had a brief chat with Emer on my own.

'You need to talk to the nursing staff,' she said. 'You do understand that they're available as a support to you?'

'Yes, I know.'

'You get on well with Johanna, don't you? You should talk to her.'

'I suppose I could.'

'Have you considered the option of lithium?'

'I've had a look at the leaflet,' I said.

Later that evening, as I was lying on my bed, agonizing over the day's developments, Emer placed an information flyer about the Mental Health Act on my bedside locker. I barely noticed it until I was packing up my things four weeks later, when I would wonder what had prompted the social worker to put it there. To this day, I don't know why she did it. Perhaps Cathy had requested it, and perhaps the intention was to ensure I understood that going AWOL again could lead to me being detained against my will. But I never read the flyer, and so I remained unaware of whatever it was intended to communicate to me.

When I think back to my situation in late November/early December 2015, the strongest emotion evoked in me now is a deep sadness at the yawning gap between my mute physical

The Episode

and mental distress, and the busy focus of the professionals around me. While I lay cowering in frozen fear over what was and wasn't happening to my body, overcome with abject misery at the possibility that my children would be taken from me, the hospital was urging me to try lithium, while Tusla's urgent priority was to formulate a safety plan around the event that I absconded from the hospital. Not one of my carers appears to have spotted a connection between my miserable presentation and Tusla's involvement in my life, or linked my unhappiness to the smell emitting from me that was described variously in my patient record as a *'strong smell of urine odour'* (30 November), *'a strong smelling urine odour'* (1 December), a *'strong smell of urine'* (two entries on 2 December), *'the odour of stale urine'* (3 December), *'a foul odour of urine'*, and a *'fetor of urine [. . .] evident in her bedroom'* (both on 4 December). I am at a loss to explain the lack of professional curiosity – and indeed empathy – on the part of the psychiatric nurses who took these notes. Why, I wonder, did it not occur to any of them to ask a doctor to give me a physical examination? Instead, the nurses chided me to shower more often and to wash my hair more frequently. I was unable to explain to them the multiple reasons why I disliked the showers: that when I had been on 1:1 observation on the locked ward, a poor job had been done of guarding the door I had been obliged to leave ajar due to my 'risk' status, and patients, including male patients, had walked in on me on more than one occasion; that the weak stream of tepid water

Safety Planning

in the hospital showers made it difficult for me to wash my long, thick hair; and that the brown liquid trickling down my legs when I directed the water at my lower body was a source of unbearable anguish for me.

As to why I didn't seek help when it certainly would have been in my interests to do so, the answer — like so much else relating to this period of transition from madness to sanity — is multilayered and complex. At the core of the problem was that I had no confidence that the doctors and nurses would keep to themselves any information I might share with them. I couldn't bear for Cathy from Tusla or my US brother or my mother or anyone else to learn this most intimate and embarrassing detail about me. Worse still, I didn't trust myself to get the story straight if I were to pretend that the constipation was a recent development. I knew too that when a physical examination was conducted, as it inevitably would be, the full extent of the problem would be evident and my dishonesty about the matter would be exposed. For all these reasons, I maintained my silence, and the longer I did so, the more difficult it became to break it.

It is not my intention here to suggest that these deliberations were entirely those of a sane person. But I don't view them as completely irrational either. Rather I see them as indicative of just how wounded and frightened I was. The elimination of waste products from the body is a basic physiological process necessary for survival. I believe that nothing sums up the total breakdown of communication between me

The Episode

and my hospital carers as succinctly and as poignantly as my failure to ask for assistance with this fundamental necessity.

Years later, and with the help of a trauma therapist, I learned to put an alternative – or rather additional – interpretation on the secret I had held on to so tenaciously in the final months of 2015. I came to view it as a desperate act of rebellion in the warped reality of misunderstandings and humiliations that characterized my experience of in-patient life. I had lost control over almost every other aspect of my existence. Other people decided and monitored what I ate, when I slept, what drugs I took, when I could see my children and even what my words meant and what my 'real' thoughts were. With the dawning realization of what was wrong with my body came an unconscious determination that this would be one aspect of my hospital life that I would not permit them to lay claim to. Strange as it may sound, I derived strength from being able to look the medical professionals and social workers in the eye and think *there's one thing that's happening to me right now that you know nothing about*. The fact that I managed to sustain this pitiful act of defiance right up to my discharge from hospital and beyond, despite the growing distress and physical suffering it caused me, says more, I believe, about the disempowering effects of the environment in which I found myself than about any cognitive or emotional impairment I might still have been suffering from.

19

Pink Armchair

Within days of the 'safety planning' meeting on 27 November, I was called into a weekly team meeting, chaired once again by my consultant psychiatrist, Dr Alpha, to be told that my discharge home was being planned for before Christmas. I reacted with bewilderment to the congratulations of the assembled team, at a loss to understand how this development squared with the proposed introduction of a new drug, or with the fact that I was being prevented from seeing my children alone even within the walls of the hospital. *'The team spoke with M regarding commencement of lithium therapy,'* the entry from 30 November states, *'however M is reluctant to start same as it is "more medications".'* Having heard my reservations for a second time, the team let the matter drop and never returned to it again.

Over the following weeks, I was left to grapple alone with a terrifying scenario that made no sense to me. I was to be discharged home, it seemed, but Tusla had told me that I would not have unsupervised access to my children. So where would the children be?

*

The Episode

Meanwhile, I was spending almost all my waking hours lying fully clothed on top of my bed, fretting over the consequences of my breakdown. I worried about my job and wondered would it still be there for me on my discharge when I had ignored sick-leave procedures in the early weeks of my breakdown. I obsessed about money and about how much longer my funds would last. Most of all, I agonized over the possibility that I would not be reunited with my children. I chastised myself over my inability in the months after John died to derive enough comfort to keep me going from my beautiful sons, who were his legacy and his gift to me. I tormented myself over my careless words while on the locked ward and over the renewed threat of foster care. And I fretted over the consequences of severe and untreated constipation. Every day, what I yearned for more than anything else was nightfall, so I could stand in line with my fellow patients for the drugs that would induce a black, dreamless sleep. And every night before I lost consciousness, I willed myself not to wake up in the morning. Not because I was still suffering from the symptoms of a depressive illness, but due to the dire hopelessness of my situation.

I was repeatedly encouraged at this time to participate in occupational therapy, uniformly referred to by patients and staff as 'OT'. My room-mate at this time seemed to be obsessed with OT: it appeared to be an enormous source of guilt to her as something that she should be availing of but wasn't. She would mention it all the time, in conversation with me, with the nurses, and with her husband when he came for his daily visits to our shared room. Thirty, forty, fifty times a day I would hear her uttering the two syllables 'Oh – Tee', like a sigh or a groan, even when she may have believed she was alone.

For my part, I attended a few of the sessions on offer in the basement during my last month in hospital. I remember a baking class during which I had to excuse myself repeatedly to use the toilet, carefully washing my hands each time, fearful that whatever was wrong with my insides would contaminate the cake we were baking for consumption by the other patients. I also recall a mindfulness session and being taught there how to eat a raisin 'mindfully'. I did not need to be reminded of how to bake a cake, or that coconut oil was a healthier option than butter, and I certainly did not need to learn how to eat a minuscule portion of food 'mindfully' while contemplating the potentially dire consequences of chronic constipation and the very real possibility of losing my children to a terrible misunderstanding.

By early December, I could no longer urinate sitting down. I would hold the urine in for hours on end until I felt my bladder about to burst, and then stand over the front of a toilet bowl as the contents came gushing out, tears of relief rolling down my face. During my last few weeks in hospital, I also experienced a number of involuntary bladder explosions, one of which was on Wednesday, 2 December, my

The Episode

older son's ninth birthday. By a happy coincidence, Wednesdays had become the children's visiting day, and I had organized through my mother for some books to be purchased and wrapped in colourful paper for me to give the birthday boy instead of the Minecraft Lego sets he so desperately wanted but that couldn't be purchased locally. Tusla social worker Cathy met me beforehand on the ward. As she accompanied me along the sterile corridors towards the family room on the ground floor of the hospital, I felt an agonizing churning in my intestines and a heavy weight pushing painfully against my bladder. I turned my face away from her, while a powerful, uncontrollable force drenched my lower body with hot, acrid liquid.

From the moment we met the children that afternoon, I was terrified of them spotting my soaking clothes or noticing the smell. After my son had opened his gift and stared in disappointment at the unwanted books, we played some board games and threw a ball about in the small outdoor area adjacent to the family room as I squatted uncomfortably and moved about stiffly in the wet clothes sticking to my lower body.

'What's the funny smell?' one of my sons whispered to me when Cathy was out of earshot. 'Did you do a wee?'

'No,' I muttered quickly and unconvincingly. 'It's nothing. Nothing at all.'

Cathy wrote that the visit went 'well' but that '*M's concentration levels were observed to be poor* [. . .] *M interacted well with*

Pink Armchair

the boys but drew the hour long visit to a close after 45 minutes. She struggled to keep up in a game of draughts.' According to a nursing note in my patient record from 8 p.m. that evening, I stated that my '*children were pleased*' to see me and that I '*enjoyed the visit*'. It is also recorded that I '*was observed to have urinary incontinence today*' and that there was a '*strong smell of urine evident*'.

I recall three other bladder eruptions from my final weeks in hospital. Two occurred in the morning, while I was still in bed with a full bladder from the night before. On the first occasion, I managed to roll up the drenched bedclothes to be taken away to the laundry before I could be interrogated. The second time, I was asked to explain what had happened, and a nurse approached me shortly afterwards to request a urine sample. I lay on the remade bed, fobbing her off each time she returned, unable to explain that I couldn't urinate in the usual way or on demand. Eventually I was able to catch a small amount of liquid in the sample jar; it was cloudy and pink, and after I had handed the jar over, the nurse returned almost immediately to ask was I on my period. But I hadn't bled since mid-summer. (Only later, a couple of months after my discharge from hospital, would I learn that this was due to raised levels of the hormone prolactin caused by my prescribed antipsychotic drugs and that elevated prolactin levels can also lead to lactation – even in men.)

When the results of my urine test came back, I was sent for a consultation with Dr Beta. He didn't examine me

The Episode

physically, but he prescribed an antibiotic and asked me gently why I hadn't spoken up about what he referred to as my urinary tract infection.

'It must hurt to pass water,' he suggested.

'It doesn't,' I said quickly.

'You need to speak up more about your needs,' he urged me with a kind smile and, when I made no response, he added: 'You must be happy that you're to be discharged soon.'

'I suppose I am. But I don't understand how the doctors could possibly have decided I'm better when so recently they were suggesting lithium and telling me how ill I was?'

'Have you heard the joke about the five psychiatrists?' Dr Beta asked me by way of response. The punchline had something to do with five different diagnoses, but I don't recall it, probably because I didn't find it remotely funny.

The final bladder incident that I remember took place in the TV area outside my bedroom. I don't know the exact date, but it was at a time when I was finally beginning to interact more naturally with some of the other patients, having previously kept myself isolated from them. There was a group of women who would gather on the ward to chat while they sat over their knitting and mindfulness colouring books, and they sometimes invited me to join them. On this particular morning, we were sitting on the pink armchairs arranged in a semi-circle around the wall-mounted TV when I felt a painful churning and a heavy

Pink Armchair

pressure on my bladder. The explosion came quickly and forcefully, saturating my clothes and drenching the armchair I was sitting on. I fled to the bathroom and watched from a distance while a loud commotion broke out after the soaking chair had been discovered. No patient or nurse ever mentioned the incident to me, but I was never again invited to join the knitting circle. The cushions on the pink armchair were whisked away, and whenever I walked past over the following week, the denuded chair seemed to be mocking me in silent accusation.

There were involuntary bowel movements too, which were no less distressing but easier to conceal. On the morning of Friday, 4 December, I spent two hours at home with my mother in an otherwise empty house. According to my patient record, Dr Alpha had wanted the visit to '*reflect what life at home would be like for M, and therefore, involve the children being at home*', but Tusla social workers had insisted that the visit should happen while my sons were at school. I was savouring a cup of strong filter coffee sweetened with honey in the tranquillity of my kitchen while gazing out at the bare winter trees in the back garden when I felt a churning in my gut and a series of agonizing, rolling spasms. I remember concealing what was happening from my mother and hastily emptying my filthy underclothing into the downstairs toilet, before binning the garment and packing some fresh items to take back with me to hospital. According to the nursing notes from later that evening, I presented '*objectively as superficial*

The Episode

on interaction, with minimal engagement and monosyllabic answers to majority of questions asked'. The entry concludes by noting that I had remained lying in bed since my return to the ward: '*Objectively noted to be difficult to engage in conversation, fetor of urine remains evident in her bedroom.*'

20

Feedback

On Tuesday, 8 December, Dr Alpha approached my bed. I had seen very little of her over the previous six weeks or so, apart from at the occasional team meeting. Sometimes, I had spotted her entering the ward or sitting in the nurse's station typing up her notes and I had implored her silently to make eye contact with me and to tell me what would happen to my children or to ask me again about my confessions on the locked ward. But Dr Alpha's eyes would remain fixed on the computer screen in front of her, and she seemed unaware of my presence a short distance away from her. Now, having first greeted me with a smile, she began with one of her usual questions:

'Any ideas or plans of harming yourself or your children or any other party?'

'None,' I smiled back, relieved to be able to say this clearly and with full conviction.

'Do you still believe that your children were poisoned?'

'No, I don't,' I said. 'In fact, I know that they haven't changed at all.'

The Episode

'And how do you feel about them now?'

'I love them very much and I can't wait to be with them,' I said.

'So you're feeling optimistic about the future?'

'Very!' I enthused. 'I can't wait to get back to my life and also to return to work.'

On the basis of this conversation, Dr Alpha wrote a letter to Tusla dated 9 December, reporting the detail of what I had said and stating that I had presented '*as bright and animated, smiling (appropriately)*'. She also wrote that I had been eating and sleeping well, had maintained telephone contact with my sons, was '*fully compliant with all of* [my] *medication*', did not pose any management difficulties and had remained as a voluntary patient throughout my stay in hospital.

Two days after my bedside talk with Dr Alpha, Tusla social worker Cathy accompanied me for a home visit with my children. As we navigated the roads of south county Dublin in her car, I felt a rush of liberation and a surge of energy stronger than anything I had experienced since before John's death in April. Finding myself in the unique position of being able to converse in private with one of the professionals assessing me, I attempted to bring the conversation around to things I had said following the events of 16 October. I didn't yet have the courage or clarity of thought to explain that I had made a false confession, and I broached the subject of the quarry edge with care.

Feedback

'I never should have said those things,' I ventured.

'You have to tell people when you have thoughts like that,' came the clipped response from the driver's side.

'Yes, but I never had the thoughts.'

'You need to understand how serious it is to think things like that. You have to tell someone when it happens. Do you understand?'

I told her I understood, and as I watched the familiar roads and landmarks speeding by, it seemed safer to let the conversation wane. Shortly after we arrived at the house, the children returned from school. They climbed on top of me at the kitchen table, and I almost forgot that Cathy was there at all as I asked them about their day and chatted easily with P, our childminder. I took one look at my sons' long, straggly hair and said I'd take them for a haircut. Cathy shifted in her seat and announced that she'd have to come too, so we piled into her car and drove to the local barber's. On the way home, I asked her to stop off at the shop where we bought our Christmas tree every year. The children chose a tall, thick, fragrant Norway spruce and I arranged for delivery later that evening. As I travelled by taxi back to the hospital after my two-hour visit home, I was happy to have left them with the task of decorating the tree in advance of my discharge and to have ticked off one item from the long Christmas to-do list that seemed unachievable from my hospital bed.

Cathy's note about the home visit runs to three sentences: '*On the 10 December M had two hours at home with her children.*

The Episode

The visit was fully supervised and went well. M was unable to tell [younger son] which day of the week it was when he asked.' The hospital entry for 10 December states: *'went for hours out this afternoon for a supervised visit with Tusla social worker, returned to the hospital in a taxi, reported that she enjoyed same, however was minimal re details'*; and, later on that evening: *'presented as somewhat preoccupied, however denied any concerns or worries'*.

Apart from my children, I had other visitors at this time whose appearance by my bedside was always a source of comfort to me. I will for ever be grateful to my mother, who did exactly what a mother should: she stood by me throughout my entire ordeal, not only moving in with my children, but visiting me in hospital almost every day, arriving with a smile on her face and bearing a bunch of carefully selected and lovingly washed grapes that I would devour hungrily as we sat in silent togetherness in the back corridor. I am also grateful to the friends and colleagues who, from early November, started to drop in on a regular basis and continued to visit, sometimes more than once a week, over the six-or-seven-week period leading up to my discharge just before Christmas. It can't have been easy for them to witness me in that environment, especially when I would start up from my lying position as soon as I saw them approaching, not wanting to be caught idling fully clothed on – or even in – my bed in the middle of the day, and when they must have sensed from the artificiality of my responses (and

Feedback

from the smell?) that things weren't right as I attempted to put up a good front for their benefit.

There was one visit from this time that I remember very clearly, probably because I spent a lot of time reflecting on it afterwards. It was during the week of 7 December, when my friend K appeared by my bedside. At his suggestion, we went to the cafeteria. Once we were settled at a table in the corner, he began to speak about the disappointment he and his wife had felt on learning of my medication non-compliance in the weeks prior to my re-admission. I sat beside him as he talked, silently sipping my coffee, remembering how a few months earlier, I had worried about trying the patience of my close friends by leaning on them too heavily. I had also been terrified that their good opinion of me would be destroyed if they were ever to learn about my wicked crime. Now, I was distressed to realize that our friendship had been damaged by information that had been communicated about me behind my back. I could well imagine the frustration my close friends might have felt on being told that I had been failing to take my medication as prescribed while they were going out of their way to support me. As K continued to speak, it felt as though my reputation was just one more thing over which I had lost control, and I could think of nothing to say in response.

Some time around the middle of December, I received a visit from Cathy. She informed me that before I could be discharged from hospital, a Child Protection Conference

The Episode

would be held. Tusla, she said, would be recommending that a Child Protection Plan be put in place and my children's names entered on to an at-risk register, where they would remain until the children turned eighteen.

As part of this visit, Cathy conducted a 'feedback exercise' with me. This consisted of her reading aloud a report she had prepared for the conference and inviting me to comment as she went along. The Tusla file in my possession contains two copies of this five-page, single-spaced report, one with handwritten notes taken in my presence that day and the word 'feedback' pencilled across the front, and an identical but clean copy read aloud at the case conference on 18 December. Reading it now, I can see that its account of the overall arc of my mental breakdown contained a number of inaccuracies – inaccuracies which could have been avoided if the report had followed the evidence contained in letters to Tusla from my consultant, Dr Alpha. At the time, it was all I could do while listening to pick out a few small points of detail and ask Cathy to correct them. Her handwritten notes confirm what I clearly remember: that I took issue with the word '*poisoned*' and attempted to explain that my original words were that my children had 'ingested' my medication and that this had 'damaged' them; that I asked her to change the tense of '*M has delusions*', as my delusions were no longer present; that I requested she take out the word '*planned*' in reference to the day I left the hospital and tried to explain

Feedback

that I was not planning anything at all that day; and that I pointed out that I had placed medication not '*under the mattress*', but in my bedside locker. None of these corrections and clarifications would be incorporated into the report read out at the conference a few days later.

21

Basket Case

On the day of the Child Protection Conference, I was collected from the hospital by my older sister, who had landed from New Zealand that morning to spend Christmas with us. On arriving at the tall, grey Victorian building where I'd had my first-ever psychiatric assessment in mid-August, we were led into a room on the ground floor and I was invited to take a seat at the large wooden table in the centre of the room. Also seated at the table were Cathy and her manager, Bronagh; Dr Alpha; social worker Emer; nurse Sue; a garda in full uniform; a chairperson; and an administrative support. Cathy had told me during her last visit to the hospital that the school principal would also be in attendance, but the conference was informed at the start that the principal had sent her apologies, and I breathed an imperceptible sigh of relief.

I cut a lonely and pathetic figure that day. I was unkempt and still wearing the same shabby clothes I had thrown into a bag the day of my re-admission in October. I had excess facial hair that I had been unable to remove in the poor light of the hospital, and I was sure that I stank. I spent the entire meeting terrified that the painful churning in my intestines would flare up with unpredictable consequences while we were all seated around the table. My mother was in attendance, but her poor hearing and advanced age meant that she had little idea of what was going on. She appeared to go by the principle that if this was a necessary step towards my discharge from hospital, then that was a good enough reason for us all to be there. 'Your sister can come too,' the Tusla employees suggested when they saw her arriving with me. 'She'll be a support to you.' I did not want my sister to hear what I knew would be said about me in that room, and I insisted to her bewilderment that she wait outside, but halfway through the proceedings I was persuaded to go and fetch her from her car.

The chairperson opened the conference by telling us that the purpose of the gathering was to determine whether my children were 'at ongoing risk of significant harm'. She then invited Cathy to read out her report, the document that had been presented to me for 'feedback' purposes a few days previously. I lowered my head as the social worker began to read aloud. I listened to a detailed account of the days surrounding my absence from hospital, following which I had disclosed a plan to end my own life and that of my children by pushing them into the quarry before jumping in myself. The conference heard that I now found it hard to believe that I'd had those thoughts and regretted expressing them in the first

The Episode

place, suggesting '*poor insight into the safety concerns associated with having had such thoughts*', and giving rise to concerns that '*M may not verbalize any further thoughts of this nature.*'

As I attempted to follow the report, with my gaze fixed firmly downwards, I heard variants of the phrase 'pose a risk' applied repeatedly to me. '*M has been unable to meet her children's needs over the past number of months due to her illness, the risk she posed to her children and because she is an in-patient in hospital,*' the report stated. '*M posed a risk to herself and her children,*' Dr Alpha had told the Child and Family Agency in a letter written on 20 October. '*M still posed a risk to herself and her children,*' Dr Gamma had informed the Tusla social workers at the 'safety planning' meeting on 27 November during my absence from the room. Now there were '*contradictory reports*' issuing from the hospital '*as to what level of risk M currently poses*' and so '*the severity of this risk cannot be determined*'. Dr Alpha's most recent letter of 9 December did '*not outline if M continues to pose a risk or not*'. As a result, there was concern that '*M is being discharged from hospital without full information as to the level of risk she poses to her children, or the level of risk she could pose should she disengage from her treatment plan.*'

The issue of medication compliance was highlighted as an important risk factor in this context. '*M attended the day centre following her discharge from hospital, however began to disengage from this service and was non compliant with her medication,*' the report stated. There was concern around the time of the quarry visit '*that M had stopped taking some of her medication and medication was found in her bedroom under the mattress*'. Furthermore, '*M demonstrates very poor insight into her relapse in October — minimizing her non compliance with medication at that time*'; and '*M poses a risk of poor or non compliance with her prescribed medication due to her belief that she is being poisoned by her medication.*' Finally, on the issue of potential risk moving forward, the report stated that: '*M's mental health could deteriorate upon release from hospital if her medication compliance deteriorates and she could pose a real possibility of significant harm to the children's safety.*'

Once Cathy had brought the reading of her report to a close, representations were made on my behalf by Dr Alpha and social worker Emer. After listening to the dire accumulation of details in Cathy's report, it was confusing to hear that I had made '*a very good recovery*', now had no thoughts of harm, was '*compliant with medication*' and was genuinely motivated to return home to my children. At one point, Dr Alpha took issue with Tusla's use of the word 'detained' ('*M was detained in* [a] *secure ward,*' Cathy had written in her report) and she stressed that I had never, in fact, been detained by mental health services. The garda made only one contribution, which was to say that there had been no involvement with the family in the past and that concerns from the gardaí moving forward would be for my safety and that of my children.

The Episode

Information was then shared about how I would be supported after I was discharged from hospital. Nurse Sue was asked to speak about her role, and she explained that she would be carrying out weekly home visits beginning Christmas week to support my transition home and to carry out an ongoing assessment of my mental health. There was also some discussion about involving Barnardo's. A referral had been placed with the Children's Charity, the conference was told, and they would be considering whether to allocate a childcare/family support worker following Cathy's continued assessment.

'It would be beneficial for your recovery in the community for you to accept the support of your family and childminders,' Emer said, addressing me directly, and I nodded my head in agreement.

'You also need to keep employing childminders around the clock,' someone added, and I nodded again to indicate that I understood.

The only contribution I recall making was towards the end of the conference, when the importance of medication compliance was being emphasized to me yet again, and I assured the roomful of assembled professionals and family members that I would take my medication. 'I am a responsible person,' I remember saying. I must have spoken a second time, because the hospital record states that when Cathy referred in her report to there being a risk of disengagement from the mental health service and non-compliance with medication, '*both Dr Alpha and M queried same*'. Dr Alpha '*explained that non-compliance was in the context of the acute stage of M's illness*', while '*M wished to clarify that she had not attended the day centre for one day rather than having disengaged*' from the service.

I don't remember how a consensus was reached at the conference – whether there was a show of hands or whether the professionals around the table nodded their support – but it was agreed by those present that my children were at ongoing risk of significant harm and that their names should be placed on the Child Protection Notification System. Cathy and her manager recommended a six-week Child Protection Plan involving weekly visits by Cathy to my home, psychiatric support in the community by nurse Sue, out-patient department appointments with the mental health team, and psycho-education for the children along with support from Barnardo's. The hospital record states that '*all professionals present were in agreement with a Child Protection Plan being put in place*' and that a further case conference would be convened at the end of the six-week period.

At the end of the conference, I was advised that I would have weekend leave in advance of my discharge home four days later. Dr Alpha and I returned to the ward together so I could pick up my bag for the weekend. We bumped into Dr Beta on the way. I recall very clearly the exchange that took place.

'How did the conference go?' Dr Beta asked, directing a sympathetic smile at me.

The Episode

'Tusla treated her like a basket case,' Dr Alpha responded, her voice icy with irritation.

That evening, I was in a state of stunned disbelief as I cuddled up to my sons and they fell asleep in my arms. I found it impossible to grasp the fact that after all the damning details presented about me at the conference and all the weeks of not knowing whether I would be reunited with my children, I had been released home to be with them. Over the weekend, I bought two thank-you cards for the hospital staff, one for Dr Alpha and one for the nurses on the ward, but I couldn't bring myself to write words of thanks for what had happened to me while in their care. I returned to the hospital on Monday, 21 December for one last overnight stay. The following morning, Dr Alpha chaired a discharge meeting, during which I wore a new top, and the two cards lay unwritten in a handbag propped up on my knees.

'How did the weekend go?' Dr Alpha asked.

'It went really well, thanks. My sister is home from New Zealand and she's staying for the next three weeks.'

'How's your mood out of ten?'

'It's eight out of ten,' I beamed at all the professionals present.

'And how do you feel to be going home?'

'Delighted!'

PART TWO
Aftermath

22

Minecraft Cake!

When I started to pick up the pieces of my life in early 2016, it felt as though a thick, heavy hood had been placed over my head and face four months previously and I had been beaten by invisible assailants ever since. But I also felt energized and, for the first time since John's death, able to deal with what lay ahead, unshackled as I was from the shock, grief, anxiety and depression that had crippled me throughout the spring, summer and autumn months of the previous year. From the moment I returned home, I slipped straight back into the role of mothering my two children as I had always done, even though I was now a single parent, and we were a family of three instead of four.

We spent Christmas day in our home in the company of my mother and my older sister, who took charge of preparing the food, while my sons played happily with the gifts given to them by our friends and relatives or purchased by me online in the computer room at the hospital the day before the Child Protection Conference. As soon as Christmas was over, I organized a late birthday party for my older son to make up

The Episode

for the miserable gathering in the hospital family room on 2 December that I had spent soaked in my own urine. I presented him with the Lego sets he'd asked for at the time and I even managed to produce a homemade Minecraft-themed cake with my sister's help (cake-baking has never been my strong suit). We decorated it with building blocks of white and black roll-out icing that curled up at the edges as I waited to serve the cake to the same group of boys whom my son had always invited to his birthday parties.

For the first couple of weeks, at least until I went back to work, I continued to employ childminders around the clock as instructed at the Child Protection Conference. It felt strange to be making the acquaintance of people who knew my children and my home intimately, but who didn't know me at all. I needed to make changes to my sons' bedtime routines and the minders' habits around food, such as serving mounds of tinned sweetcorn and peas with every evening meal and expecting me to provide an endless supply of out-of-season berries, because my mother had liked it that way. I looked on silently as they stuffed piles of wet washing into the clothes dryer that my mother had purchased and had installed for me while I was in hospital. Ever since the children were born, I had resisted her attempts to foist a dryer on me, insisting that I preferred to dry clothes naturally, but she had spotted her opportunity, and I chose to let it go unmentioned apart from expressing my thanks for her generosity.

*

Minecraft Cake!

Following my discharge, I received regular home visits from nurse Sue. She visited twice during Christmas week (23 and 29 December), again on 4 January, and then once a week throughout January, moving to fortnightly as time went on. I always welcomed her warmly to the house. For her part, she wrote in her notes that I *'presented as well kempt'*, maintained *'good eye contact'*, and was *'pleasant and actively engaged throughout'*. She also noted repeatedly that she had elicited from me *'nil psychotic thoughts'*, *'nil suicidal ideation'* and *'no thoughts of self harm or thoughts of harming others'* during these visits.

To my memory, I was not contacted at all by Tusla over the Christmas and New Year period, although an entry in my patient record states that I received one text message from the agency during that time. On 7 January, Cathy rang and apologized for having cancelled the home visit scheduled for the previous week. She paid me three or four home visits over a two-month period from mid-January, during which my interactions with her were of an entirely different nature to our exchanges in the hospital. For one thing, I was on home ground, physically and mentally, and that had an enormous impact on my bearing. Furthermore, I had returned to work on 6 January, and soon was back on a full lecturing timetable. Re-engaging with my professional life increased my self-confidence, and, when I encountered Cathy now, I wasn't prepared to defer to her any more than I had to. Her reactions to me also seemed qualitatively different from what they had been, maybe because I was no

The Episode

longer a foul-smelling, unkempt and frightened inmate in a mental hospital.

On 22 February 2016, a review Child Protection Conference was held at the same big wooden table in the same room in the mental health facility where we had assembled just over two months previously. I had forgotten all about the review conference until I came across the minutes in my records: in stark contrast to the original CPC, it made no impression on me at all. But Tusla's record of the conference shows that eight people, including myself, were in attendance. The mental health service was represented by Dr Gamma, nurse Sue and social worker Emer, and Tusla by Cathy and her manager Bronagh, along with the original chairperson and administrative support. The minutes show that apologies were received from Dr Alpha and from An Garda Síochána. Cathy reported that there had been no concerns, that I had good support from family and friends, that the boys were happy, that I had returned to work full-time, that I was attending a cognitive behavioural therapy group, and that the children were benefiting from bereavement support in school. Dr Gamma also reported that I was doing well in my recovery and seemed to be back to my former self. Nurse Sue added that there were no concerns around medication compliance, while Emer stated that I was currently stable in my mental health and engaging fully with appointments and medication compliance. All in attendance agreed that the children's names should be listed as 'inactive' on the Child Protection Notification System

Minecraft Cake!

and that the CPC process was now complete. I was commended '*for working with the services fully and progressing positively through a difficult period*'.

During her last home visit on 11 March, Cathy and I exchanged a small joke when she suggested that I'd be glad to see the back of her and I laughed back and said that indeed I would! She was probably pleased to see the back of me too. Her parting shot was to tell me that should I ever become non-compliant with medication 'again', Tusla would be informed by the mental health service and my case would be re-opened.

As well as meeting Sue and other community mental health nurses throughout the first half of 2016, I also had regular outpatient appointments in the mental health facility with Dr Gamma, who had taken over my case almost as soon as I was discharged from hospital. To begin with, the appointments occurred every couple of weeks and then, as time went on, every month, or six weeks, or longer. In April, Dr Gamma wrote into her record of a consultation with me that I felt '*ashamed*' about what I used to think while unwell, when I believed that my children had been '*poisoned*'. But Dr Gamma was wrong: I did not feel shame about having been in the ruthless grip of a delusional belief. I felt compassion towards myself for the layers of suffering and misunderstandings that I had endured.

*

The Episode

As soon as I could after arriving home, I tackled some of the post-bereavement tasks that I had been forced to abandon the previous year. I sorted through John's clothes, lingering over the beautiful checked shirts that had added a splash of colour to his otherwise grey-blue-black wardrobe, and putting his precious Wales, Leicester City and Chester City football jerseys to one side to keep for the boys. I wrote to his friends in France and the UK who had contacted me after his death, and also to his ex-wife, who had sent me a gracious letter that I had not responded to and whose opinion of me mattered, even though I had never met her. While I was disposing of John's clothes, I also binned every last item worn by me in hospital, not just because they were shabby and threadbare, but because they reminded me of the indignity and shame of that time.

I was also conscious of not having engaged with John's memory as I would have liked to. I took time out to examine his papers, to read through his correspondence with me and with other people, to study his unpublished, semi-autobiographical, satirical novel about life as a French teacher at a UK comprehensive, and to inspect the piles of old photos he'd kept of the two of us together and from the decades of his life prior to meeting me. I found the postcard he had written to me in 2001, a year into our relationship, after I had first broached the topic of children with him. He had been shocked, even dumbfounded, to learn that embarking on a relationship at the age of forty-six with a woman ten

Minecraft Cake!

years his junior might involve children, and I still remember his big blue eyes staring back at me, wide with surprise. His father had died at the age of fifty-five, John told me, and he felt too old to be a first-time father himself (all this changed later, especially once our sons were born). Now, a year and a half after his death, I found myself re-reading the postcard he had written me shortly after this conversation, a poignant portent of what was to come in which he talked about the devastating impact losing him as a father would have on the delicate psyche of our as-yet unconceived children. There were old letters too, to and from me and also from previous lovers that he would never have wanted me to read – and I never would have, had I come across them while he was still alive. But I didn't find anything in them to dismay or hurt me, and I didn't feel disloyal reading them. At the end of a process lasting several weeks, I felt reconnected to the loving, intelligent, rebellious man who had given me two beautiful children and who had brought so much richness and laughter into our lives and into the lives of so many others.

As the months of 2016 rolled by, I grew adept at compartmentalizing things. I alone knew the full detail of what had happened – even if I didn't fully understand it yet – and I kept all the memories, hurt and confusion concealed in the private recesses of my mind. I managed to park things completely while delivering lectures, meeting friends for my

The Episode

once-weekly night out, watching TV with my children and taking them hiking, sea-swimming or out for a pizza and a film. I felt changed by my experiences in ways I could not yet define, but my family, colleagues, students and friends all saw me as the same person I had always been. Most people knew, of course, that I had lost my husband and had experienced some kind of breakdown, severe enough to have been hospitalized. Everywhere I went, people commiserated with me on my loss and congratulated me on my remarkable recovery. And it *was* remarkable, even to me. Not only did I feel mentally well, but the distressing physical ailment that had blighted my time in hospital had gradually righted itself – although I lived in dread of it reoccurring. A couple of months after my discharge, I sought medical advice from a gastroenterologist who ran some tests and assured me that there was no abnormality in my bowel. Then I started to relax and, very slowly, to believe that the nightmare of my lost year following John's death was finally over. Once I was able to trust that I was mentally and physically well again, I was overcome with joy at being alive and at being reunited with my sons. I relished every minute of every day, and within six months of my discharge people would often tell me that I was 'glowing'.

When I think back to the middle of 2016, it is clear to me that I was happy, and that the children were thriving, although my older son had bouts of debilitating sadness when all I

Minecraft Cake!

could do was hold him and talk to him about his father and tell him that I understood and that I loved him. And hidden inside me was a deep reservoir of hurt at a time when I was also facing multiple practical challenges as a single, working mother to two young boys, while my own mother's health was deteriorating and she was becoming increasingly dependent on my support.

As I grappled to understand what had happened the previous year, I recalled the powerlessness I had felt during the Child Protection Conference and the extreme fear of losing my children. I relived the indignity of wetting myself, remembering the smell and the empty pink armchair, and the reproachful glares of nurses and other patients, and the fear that the constipation would kill me. I also spent every free moment ruminating about the 'what-ifs' of my care. What if I had been hospitalized when I was first referred to psychiatric services, before the evening of the supermarket visit? What if I hadn't been discharged the first time? What if I'd been assigned a different doctor? What if anyone had ever talked to me properly about losing John, or about my adverse physical reaction to the sertraline medication, or about the unwarranted feelings of guilt, or about why I said the things I said over the weekend of 17/18 October, or about the catastrophic psychological impact the Tusla referral and subsequent risk assessment had had on me?

In my internal dialogue with myself, I began to use the word 'trauma' in relation to the events of the previous year.

The Episode

Breaking down the complexity and messiness of real life into categories is an exercise I always enjoy, and so I started to think about my experiences as three traumas – all interlinked, but each one with a character and intensity of its own. Losing John with no warning had been the first trauma and the trigger for everything else. Then came the trauma of losing my mind, a terrifying occurrence in its own right. Finally, there was the trauma of my psychiatric treatment. The more I thought about how I had felt in that hospital – awaiting the outcome of Tusla's risk assessment, intensely afraid that my children would be taken away from me and too terrified of the doctors and nurses around me to ask for help with a physiological problem which, as I perceived it, was threatening to destroy my physical health – the more it seemed like *this* experience was the most traumatizing of all. It eclipsed even the tragedy of John's death and the horror of suffering a mental breakdown, because it had all been so *inconceivable*, so beyond anything I had ever imagined could happen to me. I had always sensed during the happy years with John that one day my luck could run out and that he might drop dead, just as his father had. Similarly, I had never been so lacking in humility as to believe that a mental breakdown was something that could not happen to me at some stage of my life, even if the severity of what came to pass took me by surprise. But that I would ever find myself pining away in a psychiatric hospital for months on end, branded a risk to my children and prevented from seeing them, overcome by helplessness, alienation, extreme fear and loss of control in an environment where I might have expected to receive the care and compassion I needed? That experience had literally beggared belief. I didn't expect anyone to understand why I had found the treatment so punishing, and so I said nothing at all about it.

In her groundbreaking book *Trauma and Recovery*, the American psychiatrist Judith Herman writes that truly traumatizing events have two separate, but linked, effects. First, they damage the 'psychological structures of the self' by undermining the belief systems of the sufferer and violating his or her 'faith in a natural or divine order'. Second, and just as important, they cause damage to 'relational life' by undermining 'the systems of attachment and meaning that link individual and community'. Herman writes that very young children develop a sense of safety, a basic trust in the benign use of power by caregivers, and that such fundamental assumptions about the safety of the world are shattered by trauma.

The experience of losing John did not undermine any prior-held convictions of mine. Equally, becoming severely mentally ill did not of itself tear asunder any system of meaning I had previously adhered to. But all my life prior to 2015, I had held the subconscious belief that if I were ever to find myself in a vulnerable position needing help, I would be treated with empathy and understanding by other people, especially if those people belonged to the caring professions and were acting from a position of power. This sense of

The Episode

attachment and meaning was blown apart by my experience of psychiatric treatment. 'Traumatized people feel utterly abandoned, utterly alone, cast out of the human and divine systems of care and protection that sustain life,' Herman writes in an apt description of my sentiments at that time.

I have often wondered since what the damaging effects of my hospital experiences would have been for someone with a weaker sense of self, or for someone to whom life had previously been more unkind. Herman writes that traumatized people 'lose their trust in themselves, in other people, and in God'. But traumatizing as my experiences were, I did not lose my basic trust in myself as a result. Once I was discharged from hospital, I dug deep to stoke the tiny flame of self-belief that was still burning. Over the following months, I reconnected with the core of my identity which had been left untouched by all the events of 2015, an identity that had been shaped and validated over five decades by the love of my family, by friendships and romantic relationships, by academic, professional and sporting achievements, by becoming a mother to two adorable boys, and by spending fifteen years in the company of a man who had awoken every morning with a smile on his face and, before he did anything else, had told me that he loved me.

23

Is There Anything Else?

Throughout the rest of 2016 and into 2017, I continued to attend regular out-patient appointments with Dr Gamma. These appointments focused largely on checking for the possible re-emergence of psychotic or depressive symptoms while I was being slowly weaned off psychiatric drugs. The tapering process began with a gradual reduction of antipsychotic medication, starting with risperidone, the drug I had been taking since the weekend of October 17/18 when I had made my false confession. At an appointment in early February 2016, just over a month after my discharge from hospital, Dr Gamma explained to me that blood tests had shown elevated levels of the hormone prolactin since December. Was I having my periods? Dr Gamma wanted to know, and had I noticed milk leaking from my breasts? I answered 'no' to both questions, and when she explained that the absence of menstruation was likely due to risperidone, I reflected silently that this would have been useful to know while I was in hospital, when the lack of bleeding had added to my general sense of derealization and alienation

The Episode

from my own body. We agreed on a small reduction of risperidone that day. Then, over the following two months and once Dr Gamma had satisfied herself that the reduction had not caused any adverse reaction, my dose of the drug was tapered down in incremental steps to zero. Following this, and over the course of several further months, my daily dose of olanzapine – which similarly causes prolactin levels to rise – was also gradually reduced by Dr Gamma.

I consider myself to have been fortunate in several respects when it came to my experience of psychiatric drugs during the two years when I continued to take medication following my discharge from hospital. For one thing, I was able to function surprisingly well on high doses of antipsychotic and antidepressant medication, drugs that are known to impair mental functioning. I was able to go about my daily life just as I had done before John died, lecturing full-time, running the house, caring for the children, and helping my elderly mother. I was also able to read for work and for leisure, and to follow my cultural, social and sporting interests as I had before, once my childcare arrangements allowed for it.

The other way in which I believe I was fortunate was that reducing antipsychotic medication throughout 2016 did not create any problems for me, even though I have since read that the process of withdrawing from antipsychotic drugs can be very challenging for some people. Discontinuation effects can include nausea, vomiting, diarrhoea, flu-like symptoms, anxiety, agitation, restlessness, insomnia, pins and needles, along with 'supersensitivity' or 'withdrawal' psychosis. I didn't experience any of these reactions when first risperidone and then olanzapine were tapered off, possibly because the reductions were managed very gradually, or possibly because I hadn't been taking the drugs for a particularly long time, although it is difficult to establish what 'a long time' means in the context of psychiatric medication, or just how gradual the reduction needs to be.

The main difficulty I faced after a year of tapering was Dr Gamma's reluctance to reduce my medication any further once I was on a minimum dose of olanzapine by early 2017. My antidepressant drugs – venlafaxine 300mg every morning and bupropion 150mg twice daily – had not been adjusted at all since December 2015 and I was keen to start reducing them too. I remember very clearly a conversation I had with Dr Gamma in January 2017, when I told her that it was my ambition to eventually come off all psychiatric drugs.

'*All* medication?' she queried.

'Yes, all medication.'

'Even antidepressants?' she asked, and I nodded my head in affirmation.

'Well, my advice would be that you stay on a low dose of antidepressants long-term.'

'I don't think I want to do that. I was never depressed before losing John and I'd prefer not to keep taking them if possible.'

'*Insight is good*,' Dr Gamma wrote in her record of our

The Episode

meeting, '*although very keen to reduce meds and I question her full awareness of the severity of previous episode and its associated concerns*'.

My desire to eventually come off medication was not simply a matter of principle for me. For one thing, there were side-effects. I felt strangely distant from all the sadness of the previous two years. My inability to cry – not even when my sons and I buried John's ashes in a lonely ceremony involving just the three of us in a cemetery located at the foothills of the Dublin Mountains – made me wonder if my medication was causing me to experience some kind of emotional blunting. '*Reported that she finds it strange that she can't feel sad,*' states a March 2017 report compiled by the psychosis service connected to the hospital following a one-year post-discharge interview with me. '*Feels this is related to the medication and worries that the medication is arresting the natural grief period. Reported that she felt grand at times when she would have expected to feel sad and to have cried.*' I remember wanting to experience the full range of human emotions again, even the negative, painful ones that might be required to complete the grieving process for John, and it seemed like this would happen only if I reduced and eventually discontinued my medication. I trusted myself to remain well or at least to be able to monitor my mood and seek help if I noticed a change. I was aware of what made me happy – being with my children, interacting with my mother, meeting my friends, teaching my students, reading lots of fiction and non-fiction, exercising hard, eating and sleeping well – and I made sure to find a good balance between all these things.

There was one final reason why I was keen to become medication-free. I was aware that if the trauma I suffered in 2015 was multilayered and multifaceted, then so too was the recovery journey that lay ahead. I knew that I needed to heal not just from the grief and from the shock of losing my mind. I also had to heal from my traumatic experience of psychiatric treatment, and I believed that if I could find a way to safely discontinue my medication, I would be able to remove the last traces of power that the mental health system still held over me.

When I returned for my next out-patient appointment with Dr Gamma in March 2017, the topic of reducing my medications came up again. She agreed to a small reduction in my venlafaxine dose but reiterated her view that I should stay on a low dose over the long term. When I told her that my preference was to discontinue it, Dr Gamma asked if I would keep meeting her and the community mental health nurses while tapering off. I assured her that I would.

Dr Gamma always wrote in her clinical records of my outpatient appointments with her that I was co-operative. She noted descriptions of me which invariably included words like *'pleasant'*, *'bright'*, *'relaxed'*, and *'engaged'*. It is true that I was relatively relaxed with Dr Gamma and that I did

The Episode

co-operate with almost everything that was suggested to me by her and by the community mental health nurses who visited my home at ever longer intervals during 2016 and 2017. It could be argued that I had no option *other* than to co-operate, but I was keen to remain well and to do everything necessary to ensure my ongoing recovery. Furthermore, it is in my nature to be co-operative: I take pleasure in doing things well and in earning recognition for my diligence, and this also applied to my recovery. Contrary to what Dr Gamma wrote in her notes in January 2017, I was, in fact, acutely aware of the severity of my episode of mental illness. I was unsure too whether having had one such episode might make me more vulnerable to a recurrence in future, and I was therefore open to any suggestions put to me by the professionals.

At the end of every appointment, Dr Gamma would always ask, 'Is there anything else?' and I would always smile back, 'No, there's nothing else.' But my mind was crammed full of thoughts and questions around my breakdown and the treatment I had received from psychiatric services in 2015. I kept these to myself, unsure how to verbalize them and afraid to raise them with a professional who had been involved in my treatment at the time.

'I might like to do some CBT,' I told Dr Gamma in early 2017. This was not a new idea. Directly following my discharge, at Dr Gamma's suggestion, I had attended a once-weekly CBT group course held over a 12-week period. I had found scant opportunity in the group sessions to discuss my personal experience and learned very little that I didn't know already, but the course was helpful in one respect. I remember the light-bulb moment when we, the course participants, were presented with a definition of psychosis, and it dawned on me for the first time that the peculiar, distressing and self-destructive beliefs I had held during my breakdown could be categorized as such, and that psychosis was what I had been diagnosed with and was still being treated for. During my in-patient treatment, I had noticed the words 'psychotic depression' on the personalized care plans that would be agreed upon at team meetings, copies of which had occasionally been printed off and handed to me to take back to my room afterwards. I paid little attention to the word 'psychotic' beyond assuming that it meant 'severe', and I had no idea which aspect of my condition it was describing. I was far too preoccupied with other worries to think of asking a doctor or nurse to explain it to me; nor did any mental health professional ever discuss with me the nature of psychosis or its manifestation in my illness. It was only at the CBT group in early 2016, when I heard psychosis defined as a set of 'abnormal' or 'altered' experiences including being out of touch with reality and believing things that others find strange, that I realized that my belief about medicating my children had been a psychotic delusion. Along with this understanding came a sense of disbelief that none of the psychiatric staff I was still interacting with had ever attempted to explain this basic fact about my breakdown to me.

Now, in early 2017, I hoped that CBT might help me to find some answers to my questions and to begin to unpick the knotted tangle of grief and hurt lodged deep inside my body. I was put in touch with 'Attracta', a CBT therapist whose private rooms, not far from the mental health service, I started to visit in early summer.

'I want to understand what happened to me two years ago,' I told Attracta at our first session together.

'What do you know about cognitive behavioural therapy?' she asked, and I mentioned the course I had attended following my discharge from hospital.

'Was that CBT for depression, or CBT for psychosis?'

'They never really made that distinction clear to the participants.'

'Well, where was the course held?' she asked.

I told her.

'That will have been CBT for psychosis so.'

'That makes sense,' I said, as I recalled my light-bulb moment. I also reflected on how lacking in human connection and meaningful content that course had been: everyone there must have had a diagnosis of psychosis, but we never learned this about each other, and I, for one, was only beginning to understand it about myself. As to how generalizable any of this might be, Lucy Johnstone writes in *A Straight Talking Introduction to Psychiatric Diagnosis* that 'lack of explanation of what the diagnosis means is commonly reported'. Johnstone writes, furthermore, that 'people can spend years coming in and out of hospital without anyone sitting down and discussing their experiences and their distress in order to make sense of them'.

Now, in my sessions with Attracta, I began to learn about psychosis and mental illness more generally, as well as gaining some understanding of the vulnerability factors that may have contributed to me becoming unwell. Attracta gave me plenty of material to read at home, and I enjoyed the intellectual challenge of engaging with the psychological literature and debating its content with her. Our sessions continued well into the following year. I found CBT most useful in helping me to deal with specific difficulties that I was facing in the here-and-now, like how to navigate the choppy emotional waters of finding a solution to my mother's care needs following a fall and a long stay in a rehabilitation hospital. However, I was never satisfied that I had got to the root causes of my own collapse; nor did we ever discuss the detail or possible meaning of my delusional belief about medicating my children.

As 2017 came to an end, there was one further development that had a bearing on how I was feeling: Dr Gamma had been replaced as my out-patient consultant psychiatrist in May by a new doctor, 'Dr Omega', with whom I felt more relaxed, perhaps because he had not been directly involved in my care before. He also seemed less sceptical about deprescribing my medication. He began by discontinuing the remaining 2.5mg of olanzapine, and by the end of 2017 I had also been almost completely weaned off venlafaxine, leaving only one drug, the antidepressant bupropion.

My experience of reducing venlafaxine – a short-acting drug known to cause more intense withdrawal symptoms than antidepressant drugs with a long half-life – was unproblematic. The only adverse reaction I experienced was towards the end of the withdrawal process, at a time when I was taking a small amount of the drug every second day, when a mild, if unpleasant, electric-shock-like sensation would occasionally shoot through my body, a symptom that I managed myself by taking an additional half tablet of the drug as required. I wonder now whether the relative ease with which I was weaned off venlafaxine and all the other drugs had to do with issues of what Joanne Moncrieff in *A Straight Talking Introduction to Psychiatric Drugs* calls 'psychological dependence'. 'The beliefs people have about their medication are likely to influence how successful they are at stopping it,' Moncrieff writes. I simply did not believe that I had an underlying brain disorder or a chemical imbalance that made psychiatric drugs a necessity for me.

As I was coming off antidepressants, I began to feel things more intensely, and it wasn't just sadness over John's death that I was noticing. More than anything, what I was feeling was *anger* over the powerlessness and indignities of my hospital experience two years previously.

24

Summer Dress

In early 2018, I swallowed my last psychiatric pill. Bupropion, as it turned out, is a long-acting drug, and the process of discontinuing it was fast and relatively low-risk. I didn't mark the day when I became free of medication with a party or with an X in my diary, although in retrospect I wished that I had, because it also represented the point at which I transitioned into a new stage of my recovery. Up until that point, I had Cathy's warning ringing in my ears: that if I were ever to become 'non-compliant' – however that might be understood – I would be referred back to Tusla. So it was only when I had been weaned off all psychiatric drugs that I knew that the mental health professionals no longer had any hold over me and I finally felt safe.

It was around this time that I started to listen to music again. Our house had been filled with song while John was alive, but in the years since his death I had barely paid any attention to the large wooden bookshelf containing his remarkable collection of over 3,000 CDs, which stood like a shrine to his memory in the hallway of our home. Now I

The Episode

looked for songs to help me to connect with everything that had happened since the start of 2015. I put together playlists with titles like 'Madness', 'Betrayal', 'Loss', 'Longing', 'Strength', 'Friendship' and 'Love'. For my daily commute to work, I would select a list, crank the volume up full while driving on the motorway, and belt out the lyrics at the top of my voice with tears streaming down my face.

Re-engaging with music in the way I did from the start of 2018 was, I believe, one sign that I had entered a new stage of my recovery. Another sign of change was that I was starting to speak about what had happened, and this is exactly what I did at my first out-patient appointment after coming off my medication. I hadn't planned to open up to Dr Omega on 25 April 2018, but when he asked me, as he always did at the end, whether there was 'anything else', I found myself revealing some of my true feelings about my hospital experiences. '*Tearful when discussing her admission,*' he wrote in his clinical note, where the word 'admission' refers to the time I spent in hospital.

'That Child Protection Conference was completely traumatic for me,' I added. 'They even had the guards there.'

Dr Omega nodded that he understood.

'And now the boys' names are on an at-risk register. I don't actually know what that means,' I said, feeling the heat rising to my face.

'I could put you in touch with one of our social workers,'

he said, 'although it may not be the social worker who was involved at the time. Do you think this might help?'

'It might,' I said.

We moved on to a brief discussion of the concept of risk. Dr Omega spoke about the difficulty of assessing risk, and he shared an anecdote about a patient who had committed suicide directly after assuring Dr Omega that he was doing fine.

'*She is very thankful for all the care she received and how well she is at present,*' Dr Omega wrote in his clinical note of the appointment, '*but did feel that certain things could have been done better when she was unwell. I discussed these with her and we agreed on these issues.*' When I left his office that day, I felt a flicker of satisfaction at having had, for the first time, an interaction with a mental health professional from that service that approximated to an open conversation between equals. Over the following days, as I reflected further on my meeting with Dr Omega, my mind would return many times to a suggestion he had made: that I write a letter. Eventually, I decided that this was exactly what I would do: I was going to write Dr Omega a letter about the whole appalling experience.

I devoted an entire weekend to drafting and redrafting my letter, trying to identify the main concerns and questions I had relating to my care. I ended up composing a chronological account of what had happened to me between August and December 2015. I was careful to begin by expressing my

The Episode

gratitude to Dr Omega and his team for helping to make me better, but I also shared details of my constipation for the first time, described the psychological impact of being referred to Tusla at the height of my psychotic episode, and wrote about what my 'thoughts' and 'intentions' had actually been the day I left the hospital without permission. The letter ran to five pages and concluded with a number of questions, including: Why was the story of non-compliance put out there? Why, when somebody is as ill and as vulnerable as I was, are they expected to open up at team meetings to a room full of mental health professionals? Why was it not possible during the whole time I was languishing in bed in hospital for one person to talk to me kindly and empathetically about what was going on with Tusla, or to explain to me what psychotic delusions are?

On the morning of 1 May 2018, I dropped the letter in to the mental health facility on my way to work. I remember sobbing during my commute across the city that morning. Before I got out of the car, I rang 'Rachel', the child-support worker from Barnardo's who had first been introduced to me two years previously, and who was now providing bereavement support to my younger son. She offered to read my letter and to discuss the contents with me. I visited her office later that week, where she listened to my story and allowed me to cry tears of rage in her presence.

Exactly one month after I had dropped off my letter at the mental health facility, I heard back from Dr Omega. I remember the landline ringing in the sitting-room late on a Friday afternoon, and the familiar voice introducing himself over the phone as I gesticulated at my children to keep the noise down.

'I've read your letter,' Dr Omega said, 'and I've shared it with other members of the team, like you suggested. There's a lot of learning in there for us.'

'That's good,' I responded.

'I could arrange to meet you, along with Emer, the social worker involved at the time,' he offered. 'If you think this would be helpful.'

'Extremely helpful,' I responded without hesitation.

The meeting with Dr Omega and social worker Emer took place in his office in a prefabricated building at the back of the mental health facility on Friday, 22 June 2018. I had decided that I wasn't prepared to face it on my own and I asked an old friend whom I'd known since my early lecturing years to come along with me. I chose this particular friend for a number of reasons: for her intelligence and her unjudgemental nature; because she and I had lived and worked together at the start of our lecturing careers and so had been friends, colleagues and housemates who had built up a trust and understanding over many years; and because, while she had often visited me during my hospital stay and had even taken care of my sons for a night or two at that time, she hadn't been involved in discussions with the professionals

The Episode

over their care, which meant that her view of me had not been tainted by being told that I was non-compliant with medication, or worse. Nevertheless, I felt anxious about handing her a copy of my letter to Dr Omega in advance of the meeting, and I asked her to destroy it once she had familiarized herself with its contents.

I put on my most colourful summer dress and cycled the five miles from my home for the meeting. I knew that I would be encountering Emer for the first time since Tusla's review case conference almost two-and-a-half years previously, and I wanted to negate the powerlessness I had felt at that time by demonstrating to her that I was thriving and radiating good health and well-being. Once we had taken our places on the four chairs placed in a circle in the middle of Dr Omega's office, we discussed the events of the second half of 2015. Both he and Emer looked through my records while we were talking in order to verify dates and developments.

'Her husband had died, you know,' was the only contribution my friend made, as if she felt the need to remind the professionals of why I had been in their care in the first place, and they nodded to indicate that they were aware of that.

'Do you remember the day you left the hospital?' Dr Omega asked me at one stage.

'I remember it very clearly,' I responded. 'And I remember what I said after I returned about wanting to harm my children: I never should have said those things. The only reason I did was because of the questions I was asked and because I was so susceptible.' I had coached myself to say this while preparing for the meeting. It was a point that I was eager to get across, and when I eventually read the notes taken by Emer, I was satisfied that my words had been recorded correctly.

We spent the second half of the meeting talking about Tusla. We discussed the circumstances of my referral to the agency and what it meant for the names of my children to remain on an at-risk register, albeit with an 'inactive' status, until they turned eighteen. I also talked about what the Child Protection Conference shortly before my discharge had felt like for me. To my subsequent regret, I never asked the two mental health professionals sitting in front of me to comment on the way a trivial instance of medication non-compliance had been blown up into a huge issue, or on the intimidating effect of team meetings on vulnerable patients, or on the absence of talking therapy throughout my hospital stay. If I could have that meeting again, those are the questions I would home in on; I would not allow the conversation to drift off to matters involving a different agency for which the mental health service had no responsibility.

When my friend and I came out into the mid-summer sunshine after almost two hours inside the building, we made our way to her car, where we sat for some time and reflected.

'Typical male consultant,' my friend said, rolling her eyes, but I found myself wanting to defend Dr Omega.

'He's not bad, you know,' I said, thinking of all the ways in which Dr Omega had helped me, including facilitating my wish to come off medication and organizing the meeting in response to my letter.

'I thought the social worker was a bit more approachable,' my friend continued.

'Yeah, she seemed almost apologetic,' I agreed. I had been struck by Emer's demeanour, which had seemed to mirror back to me many of the same emotions I had always felt in her presence two-and-a-half years previously: discomfort, embarrassment, fear, and possibly even shame and guilt.

'I'm happy I was able to talk to them. And it really helped to have you there,' I told my friend before I jumped on my bike to cycle home.

My last out-patient appointment took place on 19 September 2018, just over three years after I had first been referred to the mental health service. 'You had all the symptoms of psychotic depression, especially the guilt,' I remember Dr Omega telling me during the appointment. This was the first time that any mental health specialist had explained to me that guilt was a symptom of the condition they had diagnosed me with, and I was surprised and interested to learn this.

As we were shaking hands and I was about to leave his office for the last time, Dr Omega said: 'You know, I always sensed that you didn't like us.' I burst out laughing at his understatement and at the feeling of having been rumbled

Summer Dress

by my consultant psychiatrist, who, after all, reads people's minds for a living and had obviously seen through my pleasant and co-operative exterior to the darker feelings of hurt and resentment towards his institution that were lurking deep inside me.

25

I Know I Have Myself

When I was discharged from psychiatric services in the autumn of 2018, I had no understanding of what had happened to me three years previously, especially when it came to the nature of and reasons for my mental collapse. The shock of losing John so suddenly and so unexpectedly, with two small children to care for, had certainly been deeply traumatic. But even that didn't seem sufficient to explain why my mental health had deteriorated so rapidly and so catastrophically. Furthermore, while I could understand what had led me to make my false confession, I remained perplexed about the peculiar and self-incriminating delusional belief about medication and my children that had held me in its merciless grip during my breakdown. And why was I so desperate to admit to a heinous 'crime' when I was simultaneously terrified of the consequences for me and my family and when a small part of me always knew that I had never committed the 'crime' in the first place?

With all these questions demanding answers, I spent my limited free time immersing myself in publications with

I Know I Have Myself

titles like *Doctoring the Mind*, *Tales from the Madhouse*, and *Understanding Psychosis and Schizophrenia*. I also read numerous first-hand accounts of mental illness, classics such as Kay Redfield Jamison's *An Unquiet Mind* and William Styron's *Darkness Visible* alongside more recent memoirs like *Mind on Fire* by Arnold Thomas Fanning, *The Scar* by Mary Cregan and *Heavy Light* by Horatio Clare. Eventually, I was able to develop a psychological interpretation of my mental collapse and to make sense of the content, form and purpose of the self-destructive and delusional belief that had taken hold of me at the acute stage of my breakdown.

I believe that the extreme sadness I felt in the immediate aftermath of John's death, agonizing as it was, was part of a healthy grieving process. But I felt crushed by the lonely burden of responsibility for my two sons, and I was consumed by anxiety over what the future might hold for us. By summer 2015, my 'window of tolerance' (the term used by psychologists to refer to the zone of arousal in which a person is able to function effectively) was greatly diminished. Every new challenge filled me with apprehension. And the excruciating burning under my skin that began after I tried sertraline in early August, coupled with my apparently futile attempts to elicit help, drove me to hopelessness and despair.

The delusional belief that held me captive for two months from late August to late October centred around worries that had now developed into obsessions – about my

The Episode

children's well-being following their father's death, and about the potentially harmful side-effects of psychiatric drugs. The delusion under which I laboured combined elements of both fixations, and it was full of metaphorical meaning. My guilt at the 'damage' I had supposedly inflicted originated in the trauma of 21 April and the days and weeks following, when a mistaken belief took hold of me that the children's suffering was somehow *my* doing, and *my* fault: by 'allowing' their father to die I had failed to protect them. It is particularly striking that the damage I claimed to have inflicted on them was, in fact, the impairment I was suffering from myself. In my confused conversations with staff in the day centre and the psychiatric hospital, I listed several changes in the children in relation to memory, creativity and their academic and social skills. But *I* was the one who was experiencing these deficits. It was *my* academic and social performance and *my* powers of recall that were impaired; *I* had disconnected from *my* friends; and *I* was no longer able to be creative.

It is my conviction now that my frantic disclosures about medicating my children were a desperate attempt to communicate to the psychiatric staff not only my profound sorrow at the children's loss, but also what the symptoms of severe depression and the debilitating side-effects of psychiatric drugs felt like from the inside. And, on a very basic level of survival, these disclosures elicited the benefit I needed: I was re-admitted to hospital, divested of all my responsibilities and put on different medication. By the time I was discharged ten weeks later, I was no longer clinically depressed or labouring under any kind of delusional belief. My experience of those weeks was punishing and traumatizing. But at least I *survived*. And for that, I have to thank the hospital.

Lucy Johnstone writes that 'however unusual, confusing, overwhelming or frightening someone's thoughts, feelings and behaviours are, *there is a way of making sense of them*'. She urges her fellow professionals to base their work on this principle and points out that because psychotic experiences 'often express their messages symbolically, not literally, it can take quite a lot of joint work to clarify their meaning'. In my case, it *has* been possible to figure out the symbolic meaning of my frightening thoughts, even if it has taken me an enormous amount of work, on my own, to achieve this. I believe that the mental health staff treating me could have made sense of them at the time. But for this to happen, they would have needed to engage with me as a unique human being with a unique history and a unique way of experiencing things. Not by asking me repeatedly at team meetings if I had 'thoughts of harm' when multiple pairs of eyes were trained on me awaiting my response, but by gently and gradually drawing me out and earning my confidence in a one-to-one relationship with a single, trustable, therapeutic figure.

*

The Episode

In the latter stages of writing this book, I read *Desperate Remedies* by Andrew Scull, a meticulous and beautifully written study of the modern history of psychiatric practice up to the present day. The book contains harrowing descriptions of insulin coma therapy, mass sterilization, the extraction of teeth and tonsils, the removal of colons and cervixes, along with prefrontal and transorbital lobotomies as physical treatments used in the past for mental breakdown. By the time I had finished Scull's book, I felt lucky not to have been in need of psychiatric intervention in an earlier era. I also felt lucky not to have suffered the more severe metabolic and cardiovascular side-effects associated with the high doses of psychiatric drugs I was prescribed during and after my hospital stay. Finally, I considered it my good fortune that, unlike many others who have been prescribed such drugs, I experienced the gradual tapering off over the two years following my discharge as relatively uncomplicated and symptom-free.

Scull's book helped me understand with new clarity that I had been caught up in a mental health system that is sick. It's not just me or Andrew Scull or Lucy Johnstone who says this: in 2020, the United Nations published a hard-hitting report by Special Rapporteur Dainius Pūras highlighting the 'need for a paradigm shift' in mental health care away from a one-size-fits-all system 'dominated by a reductionist biomedical model that uses medicalization to justify coercion as a systemic practice and qualifies the diverse human responses to harmful underlying and social determinants [. . .] as "disorders" that need treatment', towards one that is 'rights-based, holistic and rooted in the lived experience' of its users. The Rapporteur refers in his report to a 'frozen status quo' of psychiatric treatment, which embodies an unwillingness to 'confront human suffering meaningfully' and 'an intolerance towards the normal negative emotions everyone experiences in life'. This chimes with my own experience of finding myself disempowered, stigmatized, retraumatized and even dehumanized by treatment.

While reading has been an important part of my recovery journey, finding ways to tell my story has been even more helpful. Judith Herman describes recovery from trauma as a three-stage process involving empowerment of the survivor and the creation of new connections with other people. I recognize my early post-discharge self in what Herman writes about the first stage of recovery: establishing safety. As for the second stage, by the time I was discharged from psychiatric services in late 2018, I was already engaged in 'remembrance and mourning' as I listened to my playlists of songs, read grief and madness memoirs, started to research the literature on mental breakdown, psychiatric treatment and child protection, and decided to request my records under the Freedom of Information Act, first from Tusla and then from the mental health service.

The third stage of Herman's model involves 'restoration

The Episode

of the breach between the traumatized person and the community'. She writes that some people find a 'survivor mission' and make their trauma the basis for social action. Such missions can take many forms, Herman adds, but common to all these efforts are 'public truth-telling' and 'a dedication to raising public awareness'. In this way, the personal tragedy may be transcended and some meaning given to the traumatic experience.

When I wrote my letter to Dr Omega in April 2018, I discovered for the first time that putting my experiences on paper was beneficial to me, even if it was an intensely difficult and painful undertaking. Shortly afterwards, I decided to capture the whole narrative of what had happened to me in 2015 in book form. I found myself driven to write by a strong desire to reclaim my own story, but I was simultaneously repelled by the subject matter and by the need to delve into my records in order to understand and describe my experiences. I also found it too distressing to write the story in the order in which it had happened. It was easier, I discovered, to approach the narrative from multiple angles simultaneously, and so I started to produce short chapters in no particular order, each with a narrow and specific focus. Working like this meant that when it became too onerous for me to continue with one particular topic, the chapter could be put to one side until I was ready to confront it again. In this way, a chronicle began to come together like a large mosaic whose individual stones I kept polishing until I was satisfied that they shone linguistically and that they adequately captured the essence of my experience.

I interrogated my motivations for writing. *It's for myself, so I can understand*, I would tell myself, and it is certainly true that I have learned an enormous amount about mental breakdown, psychiatry and child protection services as a result of researching and writing my story. *It's for my sons*, I would add sometimes, so that one day, they may choose to read the story of what happened to their mother in the months following their father's death. But mostly I suspected that I was writing with the aim of daring to 'speak about the unspeakable in public', as Herman puts it. I knew that the trauma could not be undone, but I also recognized the importance of letting others know what happened to me, not only for my own personal well-being but also for the health of the larger society.

Herman sees the resolution of trauma as an ongoing process that is 'never final'. While my own reconstruction and restoration work continues to this day, not all of this has been on my own or unsupported by other people. In spring 2019, I made the acquaintance of a senior psychologist in a management position in the Health Service Executive (HSE). We were meeting to discuss how the psychology service might support me further following the conclusion of an evening course for parents of adolescents. During the individual debriefing session offered to parents at the end of the course, I gave the psychologist – I'll call her 'Fidelma' – a brief sketch of what had happened to me in 2015.

The Episode

'Why don't we meet again?' she suggested.

Fidelma knew that I had embarked on writing up my experiences, chapter by painful chapter, so she suggested that I bring some pages with me to our first consultation. I chose the chapter I had just completed – about the Child Protection Conference – and I remember my surprise at her suggestion that I read it aloud to her. Henceforth, this was the form our consultations always took: I would select a chapter to read out loud for the first twenty-five minutes, invariably struggling to speak the words on the page without breaking down, and then we would spend the rest of the hour discussing the contents. Occasionally, our conversations would veer off to something else entirely, like when I needed to talk about my mother's decline and eventual death in October 2020, or about the excitement of my new relationship with a man I had met earlier that year, or occasionally about the challenges and joys of parenting two adolescent boys on my own.

It took me twenty-seven hours over eighteen months into late 2020 to recount my story to Fidelma. There was no fee attached to these consultations because she and I agreed that 'the system' owed it to me. By the end, I had revealed the entire story to her – everything from the tragic memories of the day John died, through the gross descriptions of chronic constipation and being drenched in urine while under observation and assessment as a mother, to the bizarre contents of my distressed mind during my breakdown. Describing the trauma in all its gory detail like I did to Fidelma is precisely what Herman says needs to happen. In this way, the traumatic memory may be transformed from 'fragmented components of frozen imagery and sensation' into 'an organized, detailed, verbal account' which can then be integrated into the survivor's life story.

Fidelma always made me feel that my experiences had been validated, although sometimes I found myself wishing that she would comment more extensively on my disclosures to her. More than anything else, what she was offering me was a platform from which to make myself heard, by her at least, if by nobody else. She wrote me a letter at the end which she read out loud to me during our final consultation. In it, she thanked me for trusting her and she expressed her admiration and respect for my determination and sheer grit, and for my capacity to see and take on systemic and other failings. She expressed her sorrow for what had happened to me. She described working with me as 'a privilege', adding that what she had learned from me would have a lasting impact on her professional practice, and promising to bring the learning and knowledge into any context in which she might be able to influence mental health practices and services in the future.

In late 2021, I decided that I was still spending far too much time reliving the traumas of 2015 and fixating on the professionals involved. I was quite sure that they weren't thinking about me, and I realized that as long as I made space for

The Episode

these individuals inside my head, I was continuing to cede power to them. I needed to find a way of purging them from my mind and expelling the hurt that was still wedged deep inside my body. I did some research and found a trauma therapist who, by a happy coincidence and a neat piece of symmetry, worked out of the same set of buildings as Michael, the gentleman therapist I had visited in the months following John's death – although I never physically went there again because my consultations with 'Vera' took place entirely online during pandemic times. Vera was a wonderful and compassionate older lady with a wry sense of humour. To her I narrated my experiences chronologically, and Vera used visualization and eye movement desensitization and reprocessing (EMDR) techniques to help me process my feelings of powerlessness and rage. She also prompted me to reframe certain key scenes from 2015 and to give them a different outcome, one that was better for me. The most powerful technique of all was when Vera asked me to identify a colour for my feelings and when she slowly talked me through visualizing that colour in liquid form gradually seeping out of my brain and out of my body, through my mouth and nose and ears and pores, and watching as the colour slowly faded in intensity and eventually drained away.

Ten years have now passed since the day John left our home for the last time and our lives changed for ever in ways I could not possibly have imagined even after I had identified

I Know I Have Myself

his lifeless body in the hospital morgue and told our adored children that their father was dead. There isn't a single day when I don't think about John and the manner of his departure. I am reminded of him every time I look at our two sons: I see him reflected back at me in their big blue eyes, in their towering height and athleticism, and in their joviality, wit, and independence of spirit and thought. The fact that they emerged relatively unscathed from the ordeal of being separated from me only a few short months after the loss of their father was due in large part, I believe, to the actions of my mother and also to the efforts of my friends and hers, who supported her and played their own part in caring for my sons. That the children have thrived in the years since then is, I imagine, down to the resilience they built up in early childhood when they were cherished by two loving parents who prioritized their happiness above all else, but also to my ability to pick myself up and reinvent myself after the calamitous events of 2015.

I emerged from my year of trauma stronger, more confident, and even happier than I had been before. My sense of well-being has only increased in the years since then, despite the relatively recent loss of my mother, lingering sadness over John's death and the setbacks that have dogged my recovery journey. Every moment of joy I have experienced since 2015 has felt like a victory over the forces that conspired to defeat me. I find my renaissance difficult to fully understand. Perhaps it has come about because, like some of the more fortunate survivors described in Herman's book, I have fully reconciled with myself over what happened. I have learned to regard my breakdown as a cry for help in circumstances that were intolerable and beyond my control, and I have integrated it into my life story.

The confidence, strength and happiness I feel today may also have to do with an observation hidden in my medical records. When I came across it, it struck me as the nicest and most insightful thing that anyone had put on the record about me during the entire period of my involvement with psychiatric services. '*M typically finds her own solutions to things*,' my close friend from Berlin had said when asked about her perception of my recovery by the psychosis service conducting a review of my case in early 2017. '*M has a strong sense of what's good for her and what she needs*,' she added. Identifying what I need, locating what's good for me, and finding my own solutions to things – including by writing and sharing this narrative – has been incredibly empowering for me. More than ever before, 'I know I have myself', a simple statement which Herman says could stand as the emblem of the third and final stage of recovery.

Works Cited

Christensen, D., *Dear Luise. A Story of Power and Powerlessness in Denmark's Psychiatric Care System*, Portland, Oregon: Jorvik Press, 2012.

Fanning, A., *Mind on Fire. A Memoir of Madness and Recovery*, London: Penguin, 2018.

Healy, D., *Psychiatric Drugs Explained*, 6th edition, Edinburgh: Elsevier, 2016.

Herman, J., *Trauma and Recovery. The Aftermath of Violence – From Domestic Abuse to Political Terror*, New York: Basic Books, 2015.

Johnstone, L., *A Straight Talking Introduction to Psychiatric Diagnosis*, Monmouth: PCCS Books, 2014.

Kafka, F., *The Metamorphosis*, translated into English by Ian Johnston, 1915. Feedbooks. Retrieved from: https://www.feedbooks.com/book/8/the-metamorphosis.

Leo, R., 'False Confessions: Causes, Consequences, and Implications', *Journal of the American Academy of Psychiatry and the Law*, 37(3), 2009, pp. 332–43.

Moncrieff, J., *A Straight Talking Introduction to Psychiatric Drugs*, Monmouth: PCCS Books, 2009.

Parker, G., et al., 'Distinguishing Psychotic Depression from Melancholia', *Journal of Affective Disorders*, 42(2), 1997, pp. 155–67.

Sandberg, S., and Grant, A., *Option B. Facing Adversity, Building Resilience, and Finding Joy*, 2nd edition, London: W.H. Allen, 2019.

Scull, A., *Desperate Remedies. Psychiatry and the Mysteries of Mental Illness*, London: Penguin, 2022.

Styron, W., *Darkness Visible. A Memoir of Madness*, London: Vintage, 2004.

United Nations General Assembly, 'Right of everyone to the enjoyment of the highest attainable standard of physical and mental health. Report of the Special Rapporteur on the rights to physical and mental health', 2020. Retrieved from: https://undocs.org/A/HRC/44/48.

van der Kolk, B., *The Body Keeps the Score. Mind, Brain and Body in the Transformation of Trauma*, London: Penguin, 2014.

Acknowledgements

To my two sons, who taught me to love life again. You mean the world to me.

To my early readers, Chris Carter and Jim Walsh, and especially to John's friend Steve Rigby, who accompanied me through the writing process, provided valuable feedback on a first draft, and kept asking me for additional chapters when I thought I had no more to give.

To Steve Tilston, for permitting me to quote from his song 'After Summer Rain'.

To my wonderful editor, Brendan Barrington, for whose critical questioning of the text, careful guidance through the editing process, and sheer skill I am immensely grateful.